"Thanks to its unique inter-regional scope, this fascinat
the most updated exploration of child and adolescent is
contemporary psychoanalysis. The many contributions by ᴜᴦᴵᴵᴵᴀᴵᴵ ᴜᴇᴦᴇᴦ
offer a fresh take on the babies, children, and teenagers of our difficult time.
This very accessible book offers rich reflections on child psychoanalysis."
— **Stefano Bolognini,** *former President of the Italian Psychoanalytic Society;*
past-President, IPA.

Child analysis often is in the vanguard of technical and theoretical advances
which become the foundations of schools of psychoanalytic thought. This fine
volume makes it abundantly clear why this is so. This volume is a significant
contribution valuable for all child analysts and all adult analysts too."
— **James Herzog**, *Adult and Child Psychiatrist and Psychoanalyst; Training*
and Supervisory Analyst, Boston Psychoanalytic Society and Institute.

The Infinite Infantile and the Psychoanalytic Task

The Infinite Infantile and the Psychoanalytic Task is a fascinating collection of essays that proposes to restore and elaborate original conceptions of the complexity of mental processes in the early years of life until the onset of adolescence, and from then until adulthood.

This book, led by the Committee on Child and Adolescent Psychoanalysis (COCAP) of the International Psychoanalytical Association (IPA), commits to shedding light on new developments in theory and practice in this area. Each chapter offers an expression of current thinking and clinical work with child and adolescent patients, as well as with their parents, families, and community. The complex contributions by brilliant and erudite scholars offer a fresh take on the existing body of thought on infancy and childhood in psychoanalysis that will challenge and enlighten readers of all backgrounds. Within these perspectives, the development of internal and external bonds is the focus, as well as a consideration of how analysts work in their time with young patients at these key moments of the life cycle.

With their expertise in childhood, the contributors share complex views on the link between analysis with young children and psychoanalysis with adults, making it an essential read for child and adolescent psychoanalysts in practice and in training.

Nilde Parada Franch is a training analyst and child and adolescent analyst at the Brazilian Psychoanalytic Society of Sao Paulo. She was chair of the IPA COCAP.

Christine Anzieu-Premmereur is adult and child psychiatrist and psychoanalyst in New York. Member of the Société Psychanalytique de Paris and of the Columbia Psychoanalytic Center. She is chair of the COCAP.

Mónica Cardenal is a training analyst at the Buenos Aires Psychoanalytic Association, Argentina. She is a COCAP consultant and Chair of the PACE Committee.

Majlis Winberg Salomonsson is a training and child psychoanalyst at the Swedish Psychoanalytical Association, Stockholm, Sweden.

The International Psychoanalytical Association Psychoanalytic Ideas and Applications Series

Series Editor: Silvia Flechner

IPA Publications Committee
Fred Busch, Natacha Delgado, Nergis Güleç, Thomas Marcacci, Carlos Moguillansky, Rafael Mondrzak, Angela M. Vuotto, Gabriela Legoretta (consultant)

The Infinite Infantile and the Psychoanalytic Task

Psychoanalysis with Children, Adolescents and their Families

Edited by
Nilde Parada Franch, Christine Anzieu-Premmereur, Mónica Cardenal and Majlis Winberg Salomonsson

Routledge
Taylor & Francis Group
LONDON AND NEW YORK

Cover image: Getty

First published 2023
by Routledge
4 Park Square, Milton Park, Abingdon, Oxon OX14 4RN

and by Routledge
605 Third Avenue, New York, NY 10158

Routledge is an imprint of the Taylor & Francis Group, an informa business

British Library Cataloguing in Publication Data
A catalogue record for this book is available from the British Library

Library of Congress Cataloging-in-Publication Data
A catalog record has been requested for this book

ISBN: 978-1-032-16017-7 (hbk)
ISBN: 978-1-032-16018-4 (pbk)
ISBN: 978-1-003-24674-9 (ebk)

DOI: 10.4324/9781003246749

Typeset in Palatino
by Taylor & Francis Books

Contents

Figures

Foreword by the Series Editor

The Publications Committee of the International Psychoanalytical Association (IPA) continues, with the present volume, the series *Psychoanalytic Ideas and Applications*.

The aim of this series is to focus on the scholarly production of significant authors whose works are outstanding contributions to the development of the psychoanalytical field and to set out relevant ideas and themes, generated during the history of psychoanalysis, that deserve to be known and discussed by present day psychoanalysts.

The relationship between psychoanalytical ideas and their applications needs to be put forward from the perspective of theory, clinical practice and research, to maintain their validity for contemporary psychoanalysis.

The Publication's Committee's objective is to share these ideas with the psychoanalytical community and with professionals in other related disciplines, to expand their knowledge and generate a productive interchange between the text and the reader. The IPA Publications Committee is pleased to publish the book *The Infinite Infantile and the Psychoanalytical Task* co-edited by Christine Anzieu-Premmereur, Mónica Cardenal, Nilde Franch and Winberg Salomomsson.

This book is the product of important work carried out by the Committee on Child and Adolescent Psychoanalysis (COCAP) of the IPA. The committee has taken up the challenge of presenting and sharing new technical, theoretical and cultural developments that have enlarged this important field in recent years. The editors of this book not only address questions related to children and adolescents, but also their parents, family, and the community at large.

This volume is skilfully organised in four parts. The first, composed of six chapters, explores the landscapes of childhood and adolescence. In this section, the reader will find the chapter 'On Playfulness' by Christine Anzieu-Premmareur from France, in which she presents an overview of theories related to the capacity to play and how it contributes to the functioning of role on the mind, the understanding of which has led to the development of techniques in the work of parent-infant therapy. Other chapters in this section explore the topic of the oblivious object and the interpretation of oedipal configurations in child analysis, to name just two.

The second section of this volume, also composed of six chapters, presents considerations related to trauma and parent-infant analysis. One will find here the chapter "Notes on Breakdown in Child Development: Misconceptions and Disorientations" by Emanuela Quagliata from Italy, in which she addresses misconceptions and disorientations. Using clinical material and inspired by the ideas of Bion, Money Kyrle and Meltzer, she explores the causes of breakdown in the psychic development of young children. Other chapters in this section explore other aspects of trauma and parent-infant analysis.

The third section, new voices in child analysis, comprises a single chapter, by Amirangela Mendes de Almeida from Brazil, based on a paper that won the IPSO Tyson Prize. Here, the author explores links between autistic functioning and psychic pain.

A final section, composed of three chapters, is dedicated to contemporary considerations, in particular the impact of COVID-19 on child development during confinement. One finds in this section a chapter entitled "Video Child Psychotherapy During Confinement: for better or for worse" by Julia-Flori Alibert from France, in which she describes her clinical work in child psychotherapy via video conference during a period of lockdown in France. She highlights the limitations but also the unexpected benefits of this new way of working. Other chapters in this section include the topic of working with children and their parents in pandemic times.

The total of 15 chapters from authors from the different regions of the IPA makes this volume a rich, varied and excellent contribution to the contemporary theory and practice of child psychotherapy and psychoanalysis. It validates the contribution of child psychoanalysis to the development of psychoanalysis and to its vitality.

One must be thankful to the editors of this book for having undertaken the task of presenting the findings of their work. I believe that this volume is an important addition to the subject of child and adolescence psychoanalysis, which will, without doubt, be of interest to the psychoanalytical community and anyone interested in working with children, adolescents and their parents.

Gabriela Legorreta
Series Editor
Chair, IPA Publications Committee

Preface

It is a great pleasure for us to write the introduction of this book, for many reasons. To begin with, the publication of a new book is always an event to celebrate. It is also the first publication of the IPA COCAP, a space shared by one of us (Virginia) for many years since its foundation in 1997. And the fact that "The Infantile" is part of the title reinforces the enthusiasm that we have and guarantees a great interest in the psychoanalytical community and also in all of those who work with children and adolescents in different disciplines.

The Infantile was the theme of the 52nd IPA Congress, and it has already started being the focus of many debates, online scientific meetings and publications. Even if there are many ways to approach this subject, the different theoretical points of view agree that the infantile is the source of creativity since our birth and until the end of our lives: it is always alive. This book makes a great contribution to account for the encounter with this essential and necessary aspect, because psychoanalytical work with children and adolescents brings us closer to it in a very special way. The reader will have the opportunity to become close to the technical, theoretical and cultural aspects that have broadened the field of child and adolescent psychoanalysis in recent years.

We ourselves have a long career as child and adolescent analysts, and we are convinced that this experience is an invaluable contribution to the work with patients of all ages. In the same way, we believe that Esther Bick's method of infant observation is a contribution that really enriches the analysts' ability of observation, which is an essential component of the analytical attitude.

Child and adolescent analysis gives us the opportunity to be in direct contact with their affects, with their communication predominantly through action and with the presence of their bodies and its direct language.

If we take into account Florence Guignard's notions, we can say that psychoanalytical healing is set in the convergence of the patient's and the analyst's infantile aspects; this is the transferential/contra-transferential relationship, a space that displays the human being's transformative ability.

This book brings a wide scope of psychoanalytical, clinical and theoretical topics along its 15 chapters that were written by analysts from different parts of the world. This fact enriches the volume, as it introduces the differences and similarities of our practice in varied cultures and traditions.

The book also presents the technical aspects, and it has the advantage of focusing on current challenges. Since the birth of psychoanalysis, children and the notion of childhood have changed, from the modern era until today. These changes have come along with transformations in the family model, in the place of women in society, in the models of upbringing and with the innovations brought by the technological progress. The advances in technology have shaken up not only the possibility of intervention in the bodies (parental and affiliation changes in families), but also the ways of communication, through the emergence of virtual reality and its impact on the children and adolescents.

Freud's revolutionary contribution cannot be conceived without taking into account the context in which our practice takes place. This book goes through the current challenges in our practice from the expert point of view of renowned psychoanalysts, and it focuses on the interaction that children and their parents have with the context and the time they live in.

We believe that it is important to highlight the efforts that made this publication possible in these times of humanitarian tragedy, brought on by the COVID-19 pandemic. This crisis has laid bare our fragility as human beings, the constant presence of an uncertainty feeling and the fact that the most vulnerable individuals are children and adolescents.

But we have learnt a lot from our younger patients. They have shown the ability to understand before us, adults, the painful reality of what it is to become a danger for the health and life of those whom they love. We have also learnt from their ability to play with anything at hand, to create and have fun, even in these terrible circumstances.

We thank you for this publication that brings such valuable contributions from an excellent group of child and adolescent analysts, who maintain, as we do, the passion for their work, and seek to share it with the younger generations.

Virginia Ungar, Former IPA President
Sergio Nick, Former IPA Vice-President

Introduction

The COCAP was created by the IPA in 1997, marking the official recognition of the importance of the analysis of children and adolescents. However, the pioneers Anna Freud and Melanie Klein commenced their analytical work with children almost 100 years ago.

One of the main objectives of COCAP is to promote knowledge about child and adolescent psychoanalysis both inside and outside of the IPA.

As we know, psychoanalysis is a body of knowledge, a theory and a technique. The three are intimately connected and equally important for the training of future analysts.

From a theoretical perspective, we certainly cannot distinguish the knowledge that was acquired from the experience of analysing adults, from that which is the result of the analysis with children.

According to Hanna Segal, "in particular in the last 30 years many important major advances in psychoanalytical knowledge and theory have been brought about by analysis of children - advances which were naturally reflected in changes in technique".

It is worth noting the fundamental importance of Klein's early work with children, which brought about significant insights into the early processes of constitution of the mind. She became aware of primitive stages of the Oedipus Complex and of the Superego, of the substantial relevance of the mechanisms of splitting, projection, introjection, projective identification and the process of symbol formation.

Following the changes to the theory and technique of analysis with children and adolescents, COCAP has taken the initiative to present, in this book, a sample of its current thinking and analytical practices with these patients, as well as with their parents, families and community.

We hope that our readers enjoy these contributions and also derive benefit from them.

Nilde Parada Franch
Former Chair, COCAP

1 On Playfulness

Christine Anzieu-Premmereur

Creativity, transitional space, surprise, humour, autoeroticism

Playfulness is a creative process close to a daydream that associates a capacity to abandon to the unconscious while a different mental activity of reflection maintains a link with reality and perception. In psychoanalysis, dreaming and having ideas, floating attention and interpretation, are entwined in a creative transformation. The body has an active part in child's play as action, while in adult patients, the immobility offers the possibility for free association and reverie. The "as if" quality of the analyst's interventions and interpretations and the use of metaphors help to maintain the playful quality in the session that gives life to symbolic transformation. The analyst's sensitivity to this form of expression is essential in child analysis, as it is with adolescent and adult patients.

There are different forms of play. The repetitive behaviour of the same scenario is more keeping control than true creativity. Games with rules are not play, and what Winnicott meant by the word Play is the openness to some unconscious elements that are transferred into the stage of playing. Play is a specific mental work that can be a manifest activity like in children's life, but is later on a specific quality of attention, listening and associating. That cannot be fetishised as a model. What is important is the exploratory potential that contributes to representation and symbolisation.

Prerequisites for play are the freedom to let go without being overwhelmed by anxiety of manic excitement, and the security that there is no external demand or pressure. That security allows for the deployment of a space between internal and external reality. The threat of confusion has to be contained, as the precariousness of the play has to be protected. The mind is at risk when the limit between inside and outside is lifted. Certain environmental conditions are required to maintain play: the capability to tolerate the paradoxical quality of playing. As Winnicott pointed out, the environment cannot ask the question if the play is true or not, if the object is inside or outside. The illusion has to be tolerated and shared.

The analytic setting has a very important role at offering a frame that is a secure environment for playing and free association.

DOI: 10.4324/9781003246749-1

Play gives an immense pleasure. Representing is a transformation of the object of the drives. This is the pleasure of the Ego, assuming its identity, and the pleasure of sublimation.

Play and creativity are essential to human mind. Very early in life, infants and toddlers use their motor ability and capability for displacement of representations to invent new means of communication and playful equivalence of their experiences, the pleasant as the painful ones. Play and playfulness are developmental achievements and almost all psychoanalytic theories include play and creativity in their conceptual framework.

Playfulness on evaluation scales

Playfulness is a good indicator of psychological health, and many scales of evaluations have been developed for children, gifted or not, with disabilities or regarding their motor skills, as for adults.

Playfulness is disrupted in children with ADHD, and almost absent in children with autism. A strong relationship has been demonstrated between motor creativity, flexibility in movement patterns' production, divergent thinking and playfulness in preschool children (Trevlas, Matsouka and Zachopoulou, 2003).

A study indicated that the gifted children demonstrated higher degrees of physical, social and cognitive play styles but were equivalent to the non-gifted group in sense of humour and manifest joy. Significant sex differences were also obtained, with boys demonstrating more physical exuberance, active play patterns, teasing and joking during play, but less variety than girls (Schaefer and Fix, 2005)

Globalisation and the multitude of technological changes that have affect societies in recent years have introduced complex problems into the daily lives of families. There are huge variations in children's capacity to make use of the opportunities they have. So the notion of a danger of over-reliance on digital entertainments sometimes neglects the fact that play and playfulness are developmental achievements.

Playfulness is a major pathway to adaptation. Computer playfulness also represents a degree of cognitive spontaneity. Research on the general characteristic of playfulness has demonstrated relationships with measures such as creativity and exploration and a relationship to innovation (Craft, 2010) Non-aggressive playful play is undoubtedly fun. Even so, many people think, incorrectly, that as they get older, they are no longer capable of such frivolous activity. The role of playfulness in education has been stressed for many years, and childhood playfulness has been described as a good predictor of adult creativity. The quality of Playfulness in children has been identified with numerous developmental benefits (Barnett, 1991) and playfulness in adults has shown to promote work place satisfaction as well as work productivity.

A Playfulness Scale for Adults was developed to measure a general predisposition to play, assessing four basic components: Other-directed, Lighthearted, Intellectual, and Whimsical playfulness and rating for Play, Aggression, Exhibitionism, and Impulsivity (Glynn and Webster, 1992).

The quality of home play environment has been described as essential for the early development of pleasure in play that enhances playfulness or creativity (Bishop and Chace, 1971). Play could also be arousal-seeking and rebelliousness. In adolescence, playfulness is mostly a coping system to deal with stress and group dynamics. (Staempfli, 2007)

The lack of interest in their child's play or the inability to develop playfulness are issues observed in families when a child presents symptoms. Austerity and repression of pleasure as norms in some families makes the playing a secret activity that lead to arousal and lack of containment more that constructive play. A mother reported about her own family's repression in playing and her childish need to jump and laugh with her friends, but her inability to pay attention to her own children's play. A depressed mother complained about the impossibility to join her children in playing, her mind being stuck at the home's duties, empty of any representation, becoming irritated and suddenly associating with her own mother to vulnerable to be available and leaving her daughter distressed, unable to ask for any care. She said how playing that was not available to her could have been a way to feel alive. As an adolescent, she had tried to play music as the only way to regain a sense of internal life.

The role of surprise and humour

Surprise is an essential part of playing. In the analytic setting, the surprise is associated with recovering of a function that has been lost, owing to repression, trauma or disorganisation.

In my experience with young children depressed or anxious parents, the best moment s occur when a sad withdrawn parent recover a libidinal capacity for pleasure and making links, and reports about dreaming again, an internal capacity that has been lost for a while and associated with symptoms in a child feeling deprived of an emotional bond with the parent. Children like when they gain the power to surprise adults, and the development of a sense of humour is often the signal of a change in the transference process.

Early evidence of humour based on recognition of incongruous actions occurs in seven-to-eight-month old babies who laugh during physical and social surprise play with parents, if not too high intensity, is put in the play. Reacting to incongruity is not the same as reacting to novelty that will lead to fear; an incongruous stimulus is mis-expected while a novel one is unexpected. A 12-month-old little girl was laughing like crazy when putting her socks on her head and asking her mother to do the same, but she was afraid by her mother wearing a new hat that she never saw before.

Young children use preverbal symbols, deliberate finger and body movements, clowning, exaggerate movements and vocal sounds to initiate humour with their parents. Toddler humour attempts included verbal humour such as mislabelling, verbal puns and non-sense verbal production.

Pretend play and humour share many characteristics, but differs in the sense that in serious make believe, children use to replicate real world event in ways that make sense for them. In the joking make believe, children deliberately distort the real world through incongruous actions and language, and they do not act as if the pretend world is the real world. The fictitious deformations are on the purpose of making the others laughing. A young depressed four-year-old boy was sure to make me laugh by pretending to eat all the things in the supermarket, instead of buying them, or by threatening to eat his school and all the teachers.

Play is a necessary component of humour, and as Winnicott taught us, the role of the therapist is to provide a creative space where this will be possible. Humour helps the social bonding and a relief form stress and strain.

The role of play in mother-infant psychoanalytic psychotherapy

In doing psychoanalytically informed work with toddlers and young children, the child's analyst encounters behaviours, anxiety states and syndromes that might be said to result from a failure of the early symbolisation process. Acting as a discharge of tension instead of playing and dreaming reveals that the association process between representations and emotions has failed. Behavioural problems are increasing in their frequency these days and working as a child analyst not only reveals this fact but also makes the analyst try to understand what made the child act instead of play.

The child might panic and feel distressed when his mother leaves the room; he might not be able to sleep and could be terrified of any noise, or might run around the room randomly, unable to focus on an age-appropriate task. It might be said that such a child lacks the ability to represent. A child faced with separation from his mother needs to be able to represent her in his mind. If he cannot do so, he has no way of organising his distress and anxieties.

In severe cases, it is the child's analyst's job to foster the process of representation. He or she does so by offering the child his/her capacity for representation through the use of language, especially metaphor, play and creativity.

The formation of mental representation for the baby is an interactional process, coming from the internal sensations associated with its experience with the mother. She helps contain those sensations, by offering her ability for decreasing anxiety and arousal. She gives meaning to them. The mother-baby interaction is an intersubjective process between two minds that are not equal in maturity. The affective attunement of the parents regulates the young child; this unconscious work of the parents of sharing emotions is the primary support for the infant's psychic functioning, emotional growth and eventually for its capacity for dreaming and thinking. If he is not traumatised, the child is also very active in this mutual exchange, as a partner who initiates interactions and modulates emotions. This complex relationship between parent and child is internalised by the child as mother and infant thinking together.

The process of representation is established through an intermodal interaction with the mother, such as when the tone of her voice reflects the level of the child's excitement, or the quality of her touch matches the intensity in his eyes. The mother's attunement to the child's emotions through different channels conveys both her containing function and her capacity to transform emotions. A four-month-old baby will join both hands and touch himself while the mother smiles at him, showing his connection to her. He will then repeat the same pattern of joining his hands when she leaves the room as a way to repeat the experience of having her close. A toddler will climb his mother's chair after she has left the room, and in his play will act the parent of a doll.

Through integrating the maternal presence and identifying with her maternal capacity, the young child builds up a system of representation of himself with the mother. He associates qualities and modes of sensations with the experiences of being with her; similarly, he will develop behaviours analogous to the feeling of "being together". Graphic representations of her and actions with toys are substitutions of her concrete presence. Sensations, images and eventually words, which can be summoned clearly to mind in place of the mother, are metaphors that are evidence of the development of a creative and symbolic capacity.

The early development and integration of a sense of self that necessary for the buildup of individual subjectivity as well as the capacity for autoeroticism, both depend on the caregiver's creative ability to interact with the infant. Some infants can be more difficult than others, owing to medical conditions, temperament or sensory issues that make them intolerant of frustration or more inclined to withdraw from the caregiver. The child's capacity for figuration can be impoverished by the parents' failure to fulfill a representing function. If depressed or traumatised parents can no longer dream or play, their capacity to give meaning to their baby's behaviour is impaired. "Being together," –that is, looking at each other with the right rhythm, smiling or laughing at the same time, or feeling as though one were in the same mind- are all familiar experiences that provide support for the child's capacity for figuration. Misattunement between parents and babies is a factor that interferes with the development of the capacity for representation. The typical stranger anxiety in nine-month-old babies is the signal that a representation of the mother as an external object has developed. The intensity of this critical time shows how fragile and discontinuous this representation can be.

Because the central nervous system -including the perceptual system-develops gradually during infancy, the capacity for representation must also develop gradually. The process of the formation of representations through sensation and perception requires a frame that is able to contain and organise such representations. The shaping of this frame is a key element in the structuring of the capacity for representing.

The role of play

My proposition is that the child analyst has to keep in mind how to be playful, as he or she has to keep in mind the psychoanalytic frame in order to be able to interpret. I mean that the ability at staying neutral, but warm, and strict with the setting and the frame, allows the analyst at giving meanings that can be understood and taken by the patient without being hurt. The ability to play or to be playful is also a capacity that the analyst can use in many cases, and still exists in his mind and gives him or her the possibility at being at the right distance from the patients, at making them understanding that the "as if" capacity offers children a space to express their emotions and affects.

The beginning of the psychic life is in constant interaction with the external environment. The preverbal communication with the baby helps for the capacity of representation in the child. The integration of the self, the sense of continuity and the ability to use objects in a symbolic way are connected with the way adults give the baby the fantasy of being together and feeling the same emotions. Those delicate adjustments are at risk when the parents cannot dream in the presence of their child, when some traumas, depression and anxieties interfere with the communication and make the adults projecting their own distress without giving appropriate meanings to the baby's behaviour.

The psychoanalyst observes the baby, and the interaction with the parents, tries to get some knowledge of the parental fantasies towards their child; the analyst's capacity for being playful is a free association process that can create a space for interacting with the baby and a communication at the preconscious level with the parents. The analyst's capacity for "reverie" in the Bion's meaning, can further the mother's one. To be "a malleable object" as Marion Milner suggested, is offering the child a real adjustment to his or her emotions and needs, to follow the baby in his way to communicate, and to face quietly his attacks. This requires flexibility and capacity for sharing illusions, dreams and pleasures.

The analyst's role is not only to help the parents regarding their own conflicts, but also to enjoy renew their capacity at being creative and playful, in order to connect with their baby. Playing is about a possibility for free association, getting ready for being amazed, not knowing and understanding everything and allowing the baby to take initiatives. This requires being very attentive and flexible towards the small signs of communication from the child. And the goal is not the analyst playing with the child, but the parents' recovering their own ability for sharing intimacy with their baby.

Here is a small example: Anna is a four-month-old baby whose mother is crying because of an early weaning for medical reasons that made her depressed. As she also had to put the baby in a day care to go back to work, she is full of anxieties and thinks her baby is now withdrawn from her. Anna is very tense, looking at me intensively and repressing her fear. I am impressed by this young baby capacity for containing her emotions. I tell the mother about it, and she says that it is exactly what she is afraid of, making her baby feeling lonely and being too precocious, as she was herself with her own depressed mother. While the mother is intensely involved at talking to me, she cannot pay attention to Anna who is slipping from her lap and seems to me to break down. I look at her and by chance, I exchange a glance with her; I just move my hand as if I was saying Hello to her, I see you! She amazingly answers by doing the same with her hand. And we start a kind of play at imitating each other and saying hello. I tell her mother that her baby is good at communication and very creative, and the mother holds her firmly against her breast and starts playing a kind of "marionette" play, to move her hands and sings in order to amuse the child who starts smiling. Anna then sucks her thumb and her mother realises that she could take some time at home and wait before putting her baby in a day care.

This is a very simple activity that made the baby free from her depressed feelings, but it required a lot of attention and sharing of sensations with her, while at the same time, listening to the mother and integrating the transgenerational part of the conflict.

Looking directly and talking playfully to the baby is a way to contain the affects, to share some sense of surprise, to decrease the anxiety or to interpret some negative transference feelings in the parents as in the child (stranger anxiety for example) and to offer a possibility for thinking and using words with the parents. By using playing and talking by metaphors, I think I help for the communication of ambivalent feelings, aggression and fears, and that I can promote sometimes a sublimation process in the parents, that will allow them to be more flexible and well-adjusted to their child, offering him or her, at their turn, some solutions regarding arousal, excitement, suffering, disorganisation, or later on separation issues and aggression.

Sigmund Freud's observation of his grandson is the first psychoanalytic observation of a playing in a child. In 1920, in "Beyond the Pleasure Principle", by writing about the motives, which leads children to play, Freud commented on his grandson:" At the outset he was in a *passive* situation—he was overpowered by the experience; but, by repeating it, unpleasurable though it was, as a game, he took on an *active* part. These efforts might be put down to an instinct for mastery that was acting independently of whether the memory was in itself pleasurable or not" (p.13).

And later on: "It is clear that in their play children repeat everything that has made a great impression on them in real life, and that in doing so they abreact the strength of the impression and, as one might put it, make themselves master of the situation. But on the other hand it is obvious that all their play is influenced by a wish that dominates them the whole time—the wish to be grown-up and to be able to do what grown-up people do" (p.14).

Playing was interpreted by Freud as an activity that maintains a psychic balance in order to deal with anxieties for object loss and depressive feelings. This playing shows how the child was facing his mother's absence by mastering toys' disappearance, playing at being active instead of passive, and then elaborating his feeling of abandonment and anger.

The real therapeutic experience at playing in therapy

In the Donald Winnicott's theory on playing, the ability to play is an achievement of emotional development. In playing the infant, as the adult, bridges the inner world with the outer one within and through the transitional space. In the analytic relationship, playing is an achievement of psychotherapy because only through playing the self can be discovered and strengthened. Winnicott is more concerned with the playing child than with the content of play, emphasising the way the individual uses the play to process self-experience and at the same time, to communicate. The quality of play is a signifier by itself, showing the capacity for integrating self-experience, anxieties, aggression; it has to be understood in relation with the developmental process, from the absolute dependence of the baby, to the baby being able to trust in his environment and later on to the ability for symbolic activity.

I quote from "Playing: A Theoretical Statement", 1971: "Playing is immensely exciting... The thing about playing is always the precariousness of the interplay of personal psychic reality and the experience of control of actual objects. This is the precariousness of magic itself, magic that arises in intimacy, in a relationship that is being found to be reliable, To be reliable the relationship is necessarily motivated by the mother's love, or love-hate, or her object-relating, not by reaction-formations". The magic is inspired by the infant's experience of his mother's empathy through communication and mutuality.

The child is active in the playing but needs the mother's support and sharing. The psychoanalyst's role is mostly to provide them with the space or the containment that will allow them to develop this quality in their relationship.

I will give an example; some mothers need to get a relation with the therapist where they feel understood and not accused of being guilty, and most of the time, the mother is then available for her baby's emotional needs. By using metaphors and interpretations of the negative transference, and/or by containing the excitement and regulating the child's activity, the analyst can help the mother to find her own way to adjust to the baby and to have some pleasure.

This is a dyad I know for a while. The mother is overwhelmed by her 18-month-old son, who screams at her. They enter the room in a dramatic way, she drags him, and he stamps his feet on anger, and she said she cannot more taking care of him and would like to get rid of her kids. She cannot stop talking, the child is in a rage, I says, loudly: "It is as if you enter the bad witch cavern!" The little boy stops immediately, looks at me and laughs. He takes a Russian doll and plays with it, opening the dolls and looking for the baby inside. The mother complains: "When he comes here, it is as if he finds a shelter even though he screams for not entering the room". She also takes some parts of the doll and gently strokes his hair. I says: "Finally, some comfort!" And she continues: "it is as if I was again in my grandmother's home. My own mother, she was the witch, she forgot me, and my grandmother took care of me after school, I still remember the smell of the toasted bread…". Her son is on her lap, sucking his thumb. She will talk during the session about her depression since he was born.

Two weeks later, after she had cancelled two sessions, she tells me that she would like to give the child to her mother-in-law and stop taking care of him. I tell her that she shows the same aggression towards the frame here than towards her son. She cries and says she is surprised that I could care some much about her and her horrible son as I insist for her to keep the schedule here… By the way this is the schedule for her son's snack and bottle, and she does not want to give him the bottle in front of me, and this is a contradiction because here is the only place where she could have a good time with him. She is puzzled. Her son plays with dolls, giving them the bottle; he offers me the same bottle and I play at making some noise as if I was sucking it, he smiles. He starts hiding behind my chair and I start a peek-a-boo game, where I am looking for him and scream for joy when I find him, he then jumps in his mother's lap, laughing and pointing his finger at me. She finally smiles and tells him:"You know, this has a name, it is a game, it is playing!" And to me:"I never thought one could do that with a kid". This is the beginning of her remembering her playing as a child and the recovery of her ability to play with her son who slowly stopped his tantrums.

In those sessions, by speaking in "as if" mode and talking directly about fears and aggressive feelings, I made the child more comfortable and able to play. The mother felt herself being welcomed and associated with some childhood memories, making her, after many sessions, more attuned to her child and more playful with him, who in return felt being contained and understood by her.

Body and autoeroticism

In young infants, the body sensations and body experiences are the way to communicate with the world, and the integration of the sensations, of the arousals, giving a sense of oneself is a work of linking that is provided through the daily contact with the mother, by the imitation interplay, the sound of the voice, the subtle adjustment of their rhythm. When this adjustment fails because of a pathological interaction, owing to the baby's temperament or problems, or the parental pathology, the establishment of a self-identity is at risk. The therapist can help by offering the child some attention to his troubles and needs, and by giving the opportunity to meet with an environment that understands; And at the same time, the therapist will try to give the parents some space to complain about their child and to recover from their depression and anger.

Miles is a 14-month-old boy who cannot exchange glances and does not want to stay in his mother's arms. When he was born the fourth of a very agitated family, she did not have time and energy to really pay attention to him. He had withdrawn from the outside world by sucking his thumb and stopping asking for food. When I met with him and his parents, he was completely afraid of me, unable to look at me, screaming his time I tried to talk to him. While his parents reported about their frustration with him, he started moving in the room, looking for a big red truck; he suddenly was facing a mirror and was shocked. He could not look at himself and found only my look at him, while the mother avoided looking at him. I told him how afraid and lonely he felt, and because he turned his face towards me, and was waiting, I gave him a soft toy that he put in his mouth. He came back to the mirror, and I said "hello, Miles", he looked at me intensely, and came back to his mother. While still sucking the toy, he put his back solidly against her legs and started smiling. She was very surprised. I told her that he found a good way to feel her support while having his back against her, and sucking the toy could remind him her breast. The next session, she smiled at him when he came back in front of the mirror. Every session then started with the ritual at saying hello to him while he was looking at us in the mirror.

Exploring the communication and the feeling being somebody when being looked at in a mirror is not playing; this is a real experience that will open the space for being able to play. I used a playful voice and tone in order the mother to feel comfortable and not being hurt. She could not offer her son a containment for his anxieties and emotions, neither an attention or a pleasurable contact, as she had some paranoid projections towards him. But she could share with me an attention to his son's interests and she got some pleasure when I told her that he was happy to feel some support from her.

The development of autoerotic activities in babies is a very good sign of integration of the communication with the mother and a good object relationship. During a session, when a baby starts sucking his thumb, caressing his hair or his skin, I am careful at telling the mother that her child has a good connection to her.

Aggressive behaviour in babies, or the parental interpretation of some behaviour being motivated by aggression, are source of conflicts. In many families, the sense of humour helps dealing with, they can say when a child is biting: "Oh little monster, you want to eat me, I will devour you.". Babies are not at all preoccupied by the parents' reactions towards their needs; if a mother is hurt by her infant kicking her while changing the diaper, he does not feel any empathy for her. Winnicott used the world Cruelty for young children, and some vulnerable mothers cannot stand that.

Miles, the toddler with autistic features who discovered communication in front of the mirror, was an anorectic baby. His mother was angry with him. After few psychotherapy sessions, Miles came close to her and was interested at touching her, grasping her hair, putting his open mouth on her face, and the made her uncomfortable. She saw signs of aggression. I saw something different, the beginning of his cathexis and love for her. So, I told him, in a funny way, that he was a selfish cruel little male figure abusing his delicate mother. At first, she took it for granted and found a justification for her hatred, and then she realised that I was playful, pretending he was horrible. She started teasing him, in an ambivalent way, then she was able to play with his body close to her body. She got the sense that he was not interested at hurting her and she gained some self-esteem at discovering that he had a great pleasure at their erotic exchanges.

When he was two years old, Miles was eating by himself and his anorexia diminished. I discovered his new sense of humour the day he was playing at feeding me with a spoon and I was making some noises of pleasure. He suddenly took the spoon away at the moment I was supposed to enjoy the pretended food. He started laughing irresistibly, his mother was involved in the joy, and the more I played at being frustrated, the more he was happy. That was an interesting condensation of aggression, frustration, bad object relationship and overcoming the depression, through playing and humour.

Another important point in the play activity with babies is the real experience a young child can have in an analytic office. I follow Winnicott's statement that psychoanalysts can give an "object lesson" to a child, by providing an environment that facilitates the opening of a transitional space, the playing that allow the child to go over a complete experience with an object. The object being the toy, the analyst as the one who offers it and the representation of the internal fantasmatic object: the control or mastery over the object, the playing in front of the parents who react to it, is by itself a therapeutic experience. I quote Winnicott from "Observation of Infants in a Set Situation": What there is of therapeutics in this work lies, I think, in the fact that the full course of an experience is allowed. From this one can draw some conclusions about one of the things that go to make a good environment for the infant. In the intuitive management of an infant a mother naturally allows the full course of the various experiences, keeping this up until the infant is old enough to understand her point of view. She hates to break into such experience which is of particular to him as an Object lesson". Object lesson here implies increasing the infant capacity to use objects, to control them.

Here is another clinical example: A ten-month-old baby had been diagnosed with a delay in his motor development, as he cannot stand up. His mother is distressed; she thinks she had damaged the child by her own anxieties. The baby boy sits on the floor, limp, as if being lifeless, in hypotonic condition. His mother talks to me, crying and looks in her bag to find a toy in vain. I put a shiny green soft ball in front of the baby. He looks at it, then looks at me, hesitates and takes the toy and put it in his mouth; then he looks at his mother, shows her the ball and turns it to me, I says this is for you. His mother says her surprise that this shy boy could take a toy from a stranger. She then decides to give him some other pink and red toys; he looks at her, at me and takes them. But most of them roll away from him. I tell him oh they are moving away! He then looks at me intensely and slides on the floor to come close to me to grasp some of them. Surprised to be so close to me, he put a toy in his mouth. I tell him that he is very close to the stranger. He moves away and we start exchanging the rolling toys. I say that it is fun, we play together, then when the ball is coming away from him, I say "The ball is back, the ball is moving away", then "this is like, Mom's away, Mom is back" and like that for a while. He wants to grasp the last toy that is away and fells down abruptly, his mother is ready to take care of him, but the baby stands up by holding the couch and then starts walking around the room, while is mother is astonished, happy and at the same time disappointed that he starts walking in my office! The next day he started throwing the toys away from him and walking to have them back, like Freud's grandson; the separation issue with the mother was at play, and she understood it by offering him to play hide and seek.

The process of representation

Following Klein, paranoid fears and persecutory introjects are part of early childhood unconscious life. Winnicott's view the first step of the development of a sense of self as a time before paranoid defences can be created, when the self as separate does not exist and the sense of continuity comes through the experience of "being with". Early trauma ruptures this experience and the primitive self is shattered. If this disintegration does not lead to a new integration, the casualty is the capacity to integrate a full sense of self and the full dependency on the mother's capacity for containment and transformation through representing emotional experiences. Some mothers cannot tolerate their own states of disorganisation and those of their infants. Their preconscious capacity for transforming disturbed emotions and unconscious fantasies is truncated; the dreamlike capacity associated with Bion's alpha function, essential for maternal containment, is not there; traumatic experience cannot be transformed into images and words. The ability to imagine and to think will be stunted, as will the capacity for symbolic thought.

It is autoeroticism and its infinite possibilities for playing at the recreation of memories that helps link sensations and representations and to develop further displacements. Autoeroticism as the first step of autonomous functioning comes also from the identification with the maternal capacity for owning her affects and helping the child to feel his emotions as part of himself. In the absence of the mother, the child identifies not only with her, but also with her maternal qualities. This enables him mentally to change his relationship with himself: When bodily sensations, emotional feelings and actions are experienced as being owned by him, there is a transformation of the relationship of the body and the emotions. They are recognised as "mine", after which they can be represented.

For the developing child, autoeroticism is a sort of background stage on which these images can be represented. Infantile sexuality is launched through this process. The fort-da reel game that Freud observed with his grandson and wrote about in *Beyond the Pleasure Principle*, offers his specific view on what constitutes representation. In German, "Vorstellung" means a dynamic creation, an action and not just a picture or a bodily sensation. This differs from "Darstellung" which is also translated as "representation" but means a more visual image.

Freud's grandson who created the game of flinging the reel out of sight under his bed and retrieving it, was not only physically acting out the mental throwing away of a representation of his absent mother, but also was identifying with her leaving him. Through his concrete performance of his thinking, his relationship with his mother was represented dynamically. His acting and speaking showed his internal play with the object and symbolised the absence and return of the mother. The affects associated with this process can change perception, so in his mind the child transform, deny or neglect external reality.

The roots of the capacity for representation are strongly linked with affect. The affect is the part of the drives that is the most difficult to transform, and is therefore associated with primitive defences. In the case of early trauma, violent affect will be discharged and could destabilise the psyche and its ability for representation and symbolisation. Early defences such as splitting, denial, decathexis, expulsion of mental content or the mind from the body, somatic reactions and foreclosure will then interfere with some representational processes. When dealing with these primitive defences, the analyst uses affect to get close to the patient, as affects are traces of early events. Countertransference is the best tool to learn about the patient's experience.

The role of language is essential as the link between affects and representations. All mediations are useful as they offer a space that cans serve to open up transitional functioning. A new dimension in the relationship is promoted when a third person is integrated in the too-close/too-far-away dyadic object relationship. As Andre Green (1972) reminded us, the analyst's work is to offer representations through metaphors: These metaphors were understood as unconsciously suggested by the patient before articulated by the analyst. During sessions, babies are wonderful partners who use the setting spontaneously if they are not too depressed or withdrawn. The discoveries and experiences that they made in the room are organisers for their psyche.

Toddlers and young children in psychoanalytic psychotherapy learn to contain their fears. Now, kids play video games and experience virtual reality. For some, this is a big help that offers pictures and representations of their monsters, but for most of them, this is the cause of a repetitive and vain quest for symbolisation. Playing with a young child in a psychotherapy session is providing a new experience of connection with the fantasy world without danger and helping to create a kind of dictionary of its own monsters that could be then described, told to the others and mastered. Playing or being ready to play and talking with a sense of humour is offering a child an experience of feeling being omnipotent over the world, having a control and not being passive anymore, it is giving him or her the possibility to get some magic that is so essential to keep the sense of being alive and full with hope in the future!

References

Anzieu, D. 1985. *The Skin Ego*. Yale University Press.

Anzieu-Premmereur, C. 2013. The process of representation in early childhood. In: *The Work of Figurability*. Eds. Howard Levine, Gail Reed, Dominique Scarfone. Routledge, pp. 240–254.

Anzieu-Premmereur, C. 2016. Peter, the Child Who Could not dream, in Psychoanalytic Work with the Dreams of Children: The Forgotten Royal Road. Eds Christine Anzieu-Premmereur, Denia Barrett and Ruth Karush, April, *Psychoanalytic Inquiry*, 231–238.

Anzieu-Premmereur, C. 2017. Attacks on Linking in Parents of Young Disturbed Children. In: *Catalina Bronstein On Bion's Attacks on Linking*, Karnac, pp. 103–123.

Anzieu-Premmereur, C. 2017. Perspectives on the Body Ego and Mother-Infant Interactions. I've Got You Under My Skin. In *A Psychoanalytic Exploration of the Body in Today's World: On the Body*. Eds Vaia Tsolas and Christine Anzieu-Premmereur, Routledge, pp. 89–99.

Barnett, L.A. (2007). The nature of playfulness in young adults. *Personality and individual differences*, 43(4), 949–958.

Bick, E. 1968. The experience of the Skin in Early Objects Relations. *International. Journal of Psychoanalysis*, 49, 484–486.

Bion, W.R. 1970. Attention and interpretation. In: *Seven Servants*, New York, Aronson.

Bishop, D.W. and Chace, C.A. (1971). Parental conceptual systems, home play environment, and potential creativity in children. *Journal of Experimental Child Psychology*, 12(3), 318–338.

Craft, A. 2010. *Creativity and Education Futures: Learning in a Digital Age*. Trentham Books Ltd.

Freud, S. 1914. *Remembering, Repeating and Working Through*, S.E.12.

Freud, S. 1920. *Beyond the pleasure principle*, S.E. 18., 14–17.

Gergely, G. and Watson, J.S. 1996. The Social Biofeedback Theory Of Parental Affect-Mirroring. *International Journal of Psycho-Analysis*, 77: 1181–1212.

Glynn, M.A. and Webster, J. (1992). The adult playfulness scale: An initial assessment. *Psychological reports*, 71(1), 83–103.

Green A. 1972 The Analyst, Symbolization and Absence. In: *On Private Madness*. IUP.

Klein, M. 1952. Some theoretical conclusions regarding the emotional life of the infant. In: *Developments in Psychoanalysis*, London, Hogarth Press, pp. 198–236.

Lacan, J. 1949. The mirror stage as formative function of the I as revealed in psychoanalytic experience. In *Ecrits: A selection* (Trans. Alan Sheridan), London, Tavistock, 1977, 1–7.

Milner, M. 1957. *On Not Being Able to Paint*. IUP.

Ogden, T. 2004. On Holding and Containing, Being and Dreaming. *International Journal of Psychoanalysis*, Vol. 65, 1349–1364.

Roussillon, R. 2011 *Primitive agony and its symbolization*. IPA Karnac.

Schaefer, C. and Fix, G.A. 2005. Note on psychometric properties of playfulness scales with adolescents. *Psychological reports*, 96(3_suppl), 993–994.

Shuttleworth, J. (1989). Psychoanalytic theory and infant development. In: *Closely Observed Infants*, eds L. Miller, M.E. Rustin, M.J. Rustin and J. Shuttleworth, London, Duckworth, 22–51.

Staempfli, M.B. (2007). Adolescent playfulness, stress perception, coping and well being. *Journal of Leisure Research*, 39(3), 393–412.

Trevlas, E., Matsouka, O. and Zachopoulou, E. (2003). Relationship between playfulness and motor creativity in preschool children. *Early Child Development and Care*, 173(5), 535–543.

Winnicott, D.W. 1953. Transitional objects and Transitional Phenomena- A Study of the First Not- Me Possession. *International Journal of Psychoanalysis*, 34, 89–97.

Winnicott, D.W. 1967. *The Location of Cultural Experience, in Playing and Reality*, London, Tavistock, 1971.

Winnicott, D.W. 1971. Mirror-Role of Mother and Family in Child Development. In *Playing and Reality*, Penguin Books, pp.101–111.

2 The Shifting Boundaries of Intimate Psychic Spaces In Childhood and Adolescence

Julie Augoyard

Introduction

It is now obvious that our occidental postmodern societies are attending an epistemological shift. The increasing practices resorted to technology, connective logic and virtual relationships are both the signs and consequences of a different mode of interactions. The new collective representations arising in the social and cultural fields, testify that the boundaries of the Self are questioned, extended, opened, deconstructed. Such are the changing representations linked to the emergent questions at stake in the process of building a subjective intimacy: gender, sexualities, new parenthoods. The construction and the functioning of intimate spaces, on which the psyche growths, is founded on the intimacy between two bodies. To what extend do the profound social-cultural changes affect this construction of intimacy leading to subjectivity during childhood and adolescence?

Childhood and adolescence are the crossroads to a vivid creativity, temporal and spatial experiences: a drives tank, the "cauldron of subjectivation" reviving or renewing all life long in a dynamic way. The analysts know that a paradox derives from the synchronic and diachronic double link between childhood and adolescence. The one follows the other; they share the same ground. But they also stand in a dialectical movement through the "après-coup" process. They both have their own idiomatic tongue; a different terminology belongs to each in the psychoanalytical field. Yet I chose to set them altogether, in an epistemological perspective, since an unprecedented cultural gap severs them from their genitors and the previous generations; their social and somehow perhaps psychic delineations tend to blur.

Since in each of their processes, though differently, the shift of the boundaries is structural, what kind of new parameters does this changing world bring out and impose within and on the borders of the Self? Are we psychoanalysts prepared to face the encounter with different kind of intimate spaces that show up in our patients, and during the intimate analytical process with children and adolescents? Are these shifting borders changing the paradigm of the infantile sexuality?

DOI: 10.4324/9781003246749-2

I Ground and boundaries of intimate psychic spaces: vicissitudes and changes

The archaic and primitive experiences that occur in the relation with the primal object draw the outlines of an ego skin-envelope. The boundaries of the self are constantly shifting during childhood, and then adolescence. The task of internalising a cover and container for the self to develop is submitted to the demands of the constant drives pressure, while spatial and temporal realities unfold. The topic and economic handlings of the id-ego-superego instances, ego ideals, internal-external objects balance, contribute to the past-present-future identities fit in with representations of subjective places. The bodily image, which can hold together the surfaces and the sphincters with the integrated erotogenic zones, will be disorganised when puberty comes. Drives push will be calling again for rigid primal defences touching the ego and the object (splitting-and-idealisation, disavowal, projective identification). Meanwhile, the fluidity of the identifications during adolescence allows more suppleness to discriminate among the "infantile structures" (Meltzer, 1988). But because of the defused drives, bodily confusion threats at the door since a secure space is still lacking to contain the differentiations (internal-external, infantile-adult, good-bad, feminine-masculine…), to explore the auto-erotism (masturbation) and to make the part between sexual love and sadism. Since the drives impose themselves as a concept on the borders of the soma and the psyche (Freud, 1915), the field of the body is the first concerned with the psychic boundaries.

The bodily intimacy: boundaries for an aesthetic space to grow or a secret space to hide?

The construction of intimacy weaves in the sensoriality and the aesthetic experiences of the primary maternal space, rooting the intimate identity in the sonic mother-tongue (Kelly-Lainé, 2017) altogether with the pre-symbolic language. Meltzer (1988) proposed in a very "poïetic" version, a theoretical construction of the aesthetic encounter between the primal object and the new-born that will shape the first shape of the future self boundaries. Overwhelmed by the sensorial stimuli coming from the beauty of his mother, the new-born's experiences an emotional catastrophic situation. The encounter with an elusive object, an altogether lost and present "unknown", calls a central depressive pain, as well as it arouses a question that will potentially promote the thought and the epistemophilic drive: "Is it as beautiful inside than outside?" The reciprocity of the aesthetic encounter between the *infans* and his/her mother is requisite for the creation of a passionate intimacy.

The distinction between a private intimate space and a secret one lies in the different modality of drive cathexis: an object cathexis or a narcissistic one. According to Meltzer, the intimate space stems for the promotion of love for the object and the preservation of the ethical values of the self and its beloved objects. Whereas the secret space is ruled by an omnipotent control over the self and the objects, disavowing the loss and pain that love can involve. The capability to open up to new experiences that could be introjected in a private nourishing space is then disallowed. At stake is the availability and disposition of the environment/object to share a mutual emotional time-space, although non-symmetric, with the undifferentiated and immature ego of the *infans*. As Meltzer conceives it, the secret space is enclosed and hinders the normal "psychic breathing" (projective identification), this in-and-out fruitful communication with the external objects. Consequently, a hidden secretive space will pervert, distort or obstruct the conception and the further encounter with real "otherness" that could sustain a meaningful experience for the subject. This conception ties with Masud Khan's idea of "secretiveness" as the distortion of the private space (1983), whereas he views the secret space as a potential creative private space.

Despite this terminological debate, we should give the secret an extending meaning. Indeed, the quest for a secret garden/place, as a synonymous of intimacy, might be the explicit claim of any children and teenagers of our occidental societies. This demand binds the urgent need of the (very) young individual for privacy to his/her use of the connective devices that has now become the identity marker of the young generations. On another level, sexualised patterns are hyper exposed and shown in great confusion as for to define the modal function (feminine-masculine, active-passive, etc.) or the ontological quality (what it is to be a girl/boy). Secret(ive) intimate content can be overexposed in a secret(ive) place that might contribute to the confused meaning of *alterity*.

When intimate spaces open to otherness: a new configuration of alterity or the return of the split?

The opening to otherness depends on the good crossing from the "primary maternal space" to the "primary feminine space" (Guignard, 1996, 2019) for both sexes. During the establishment of the former, the infant's nascent drives are brought to contain and cathex the unknown qualities of the enigmatic aesthetic object, thanks to the maternal capacity of reverie (Bion). The primary feminine space sets the way out to the exclusive dyad mother-child, conducting the infant to identify to the mother and to her drive organisation that contends a third object, the other's other. The function of the phantasmatic father—the protective, cleaning, feeding and separating attributes and contents of the penis/testicules-in-the-mother (Klein)—is to offer a shield against the hostile internal and external attacks, to rule the entrance and exit of the internal mother's spaces, from the beauty of which the child must be protected; the function of the symbolic father (the metaphor of the father's name, Lacan) guarantees the prohibition of incest, the inscription of the child among the generations, the entrance in the symbolic world made of verbal language. Experiences of absence and loss of the object settle there, as the conflict between love and hate towards this first object spreads. The alternative and counterpart for the infant is to turn towards "a new object in a new way" (Guignard, 2019). What is finally at stake in the aesthetic conflict, thanks to the building of boundaries for an internal and an external space, is the capability to open to *otherness*, however painful, overwhelming and strange this alterity might be.

When childhood delineates the intimate boundaries, adolescence is re-questioning the intimate places where to become a subject included in his own social-individual history (Aulagnier) by exploring their boundaries and *alter* them. A second time is indeed given to human sexuality or a second "central anthropologic situation", as Philippe Gutton proposes (2014) referring to J. Laplanche. But the Freudian conception of the interactive "two-times movements " (Nachträglichkeit) of shaping an intimacy from childhood to adolescence might be re-considered in the light of what is being now observed[1]: latency tends to vanish in favour of an extended and confused period of sexualised overexcitement. The desexualisation that characterises this moment dedicated to sublimations and new cathexis (aim-inhibited drives) is on his way to be progressively bypassed. Children seem to share the same anxieties bond to the demanding drive imperatives of the eldest affected by the "Pubertal" (Gutton, 2013), even if the mind goes in front of the body, simulating (aping) the sexuality of the teenagers. Jointly, the Oedipal nodal structure as a *complex* could be disappearing as well (Guignard, 2015, 2019).

From an intra-psychic perspective, its constitution and resolution might be rattled by several spatial and temporal confusions fading the impact of the "après-coup", questioning the post-oedipus identifications and the second repression. The boundaries that keep safe from forbidden incestuous fantasies are fading while the introjection of aim-inhibited drives and sublimation are endangered. From the inter-subjective and social perspective of our civilisation, the hardly bearable postponement and frustration not to achieve one's wish puts the marker on the side of the immediate satisfaction of the need and the discharge, according to the pleasure principle. Splitting, disavowal and foreclosure tend to replace repression and useful inhibition. The social containment is being shattered by the cultural loss of a cohesive collective ideal; the ideal ego seems to prevail instead of the ego ideal. Are we not facing the *return of the split* instead of the repressed?

These hypotheses could be connected with the new parental constellations, new artificial modes of procreation (AMP) and new representations of sexuality and gender. According to the binary and dialectical logics ruling our civilisation, the biological, supported by the technological progress, is split from the cultural and the symbolic order. The latter is tied to the rhetorical means of the "performative", and the banner of the "all-language" supporters, such as for the gender studies; while the "all-biological" sets on the adversary side of the Nature (although culturally reconstructed). This split position induces some confusion in the differences of generations and sexes, albeit differences are forced in categories erected like fetishes and idols. Surely we witness an unprecedented blurring of the cultural and social differences between the children and the teenagers, who are melted together in new categories determined by the liberal and economic logics supported by technology. They both are born in the world of computer science, share the same connective devices and often experience the same contents in virtual games and social networks.

What should we learn from this epistemological change concerning the difference and its enigma, which remain the bedrock of humanity and psychoanalysis? A new enigma of differences aroused by the changes of mental paradigms provokes the anguish of uncertainty, looks like an "unthinkable" and calls for words to be apprehended. An *"other otherness"* is perhaps showing up, challenging our capacity to really experience what the unfamiliar unknown is calling for, such as the pandemic did. Are the boundaries of psychic intimate spaces going to locate in an *"extra-territorial"* yet unknown zone of the mind? Another space whose frontier would neither firmly be establishing the traffic between the unconscious and the preconscious nor clearly between the inside and the outside. Following such a vertex, the "contact barrier" (Bion) is produced by the dream-like thoughts while creating-splitting the unconscious/conscious elements, might provide an operative concept, since it views the border like a moving, porous *bond-in-between* which can distribute and deal with reversible transient elements. It can also reverse to its negative function, generating destructive hyperbolic "anti-places". As Derrida reminds it, referring to Plato's *Pharmacon*: any remedy contains its poison and vice versa. As childhood and adolescence are the time-space for structural handlings and reshufflings of the self boundaries, they both appears as the paradigmatic shapes of bond-in-between towards new borders.

II Violence and creativity of new borders for otherness

Limits of intimacy, intimacy at the limits

Green's work stressed for some time now (1990), that the " pathologies of the borders " are more than ever our contemporary clinic. Creating supple borders like psychic sphincters is a necessary task, in order to modulate and secure the reciprocal projective-introjective traffic with the objects of the inner and external world. To find and elaborate the symbolic potentiality of otherness requires the distance of the separated "sumbolon" and borders in-and-out. Correlative to intimacy, creativity plays a crucial part in the matter. In this respect, a still precious theoretical model to refer to is the transitional space (Winnicott), thanks to which, in the path from "subjective" relation to "objective" one, the most intimate true part of the self finds the potential means to develop and strengthens. Deprived from an illusionary space that has to be carried by the primal object, the self has to resort to a defensive solution, finding a forced, false, traumatic superficial kind of "over-skin" envelop (Bick) similarly to the "auto-narcissistic splitting" (Ferenczi) that delineates a violent unnatural separation. According to Meltzer, violence consists in "an intrusion in the private space without permission" (Meltzer, 1987, 89–90). The large and consensual debate about the consent has become the shared concern of numerous teenagers around the world, as violence against oppressed categories calls for a deconstruction of cultural boundaries. The major topic on which our postmodern societies are bending over could be consolidating, protecting, creating transitional spaces that shape borders in-and-out. Whereas the mere destruction of the borders does not allow any creative experience of intimacy through a symbiotic blurring of the limits, out of which new shapes could arise; this transitional illusionary experience is possible on condition a protective shield with borders is provided, such as the ego-skin (Anzieu), or the contact-barrier.

Since the modern partition public/private does not prevail any more, a new kind of "social intimacy" has appeared in our postmodern society sustained by the globalisation (Côté, 2011). In a world where a person is "an atom in an indeterminate mass", whereas the "equality of the persons" would paradoxically require making differentiations, the anonymous undifferentiated individual has to search for the marks of his/her "auto-determination". Childhood and adolescence are in front line in this new paradoxical configuration: the child/adolescent should build his/her intimacy (borders) and claim for alterity and difference in a confused anonymous mass. Our post-gender civilisation is blurring sexual anatomic determinations proportionally to the variety of often confusing proposals for an over-determined gendered identity or for auto/pro-creative new means. In this "Faustian" (Moreno, 2019) context, the young individuals feels the urge to find a remarkable singularity of his own that would make the difference, take a distance from the confused singularities.

Intimacy in the times of computer science and cyberspace

Among the different uses that the computer science allows, those mostly seized by children and adolescents should be distinguished: animation and artificial intelligence (games) on the one hand, or social networks (applications such as Instagram, Snapchat, Messenger, Twitter…) on the other. In the former, the simulation of the original reality pretends to replace it, or reversely an invented reality based on imaginary settings shows a world made of dream-like delusion. In the later, the protagonists and the setting negotiate with the reality of human communication, its factor of distance—that is, with the dialectic between perceptive and/or symbolic absence-presence of the other—bond with the self-image. We should add to these uses, the search for information, considerably increasing the opportunities for a wider knowledge and promoted by the epistemophilic drive ("K" drive for Bion) in the best case.

To what extend the contact with the connective world would enlarge, deepen, foster a creative intimate space, promote the drive cathexis on their path to tempered object relations and sublimated objects, or rather reduce, constraint, distort, debar, pervert them? Children are exposed to screens and to the virtual world at an early age. Many scientific researchers agree to acknowledge and try to prevent[2] the damages caused, not only on the brain, but also on the psychic construction of subjectivity. Passivity, excessive manic excitement, hyper-agitation, lack of affective and cognitive availability to the learning (ADHD, DAMP), intolerance to frustration and to postponement or psychosomatic manifestations, … are some of the raising symptoms against what is bond to loss and depressive experiences. In the landscape of contemporary psychopathologies, those of introjection, projection, dependence, addiction and acting out (agieren) or repudiation (Verwerfung) and evacuation seem to prevail.

The computer specialist Pr. Gerard Berry assumes a radical perspective[3] about the cognitive change generated by the computer science. Almost every object of our daily life is affected by computer science and connective logic. They have put the world upside-down and initiated a new era of cognitive logic of the mind. The reasoning and the action on the *information*, a revolutionary element added by computer science, are quite different from those of the mental pattern of the 20th century, standing by the triptych composed of material/energy/waves. The structure and treatment of connective data has now reached a high complexity that exposes humanity to an overload and to crisis (Bronner, 2020). According to the neurologist Lionel Naccache (2020), the architecture of a complex system of data had been first following a "top-down" functioning in our industrialised civilisations; a scientific hierarchy (the head) sending the data to those who were less skilled for abstract conceptualisation (the body). In the best case, some guarantee was ensured for substantial and enlightened information; in the worse, this authoritarian organisation turned to a split selective oligarchy. Our civilisation now faces a "bottom-up" processing of information, drawing a new landscape where supplies and demands share the same indiscriminate level. Moreover, since the algorithms have taken the lead on behalf of many economical-political strategies, human capacity for conceptualisation and symbolisation might be partly jeopardised. Fortunately, the human brain still needs to give a subjective meaning to its perception, adds Naccache.

Quoting Melvin Kranzberg, Alessandra Lemma (2015) reminds that: "Technology is neither good nor bad". We therefore should suppose that the alternatives offered to and seized by childhood and adolescence also lie in the technological perspectives that make them *"alter-natives"* coming from another world and creating another one. To be optimistic, this inevitable perspective must fulfil some conditions of possibility that deal with intimacy.

Serge Tisseron (2007, 2011) proposed to categorise a new kind of intimate space which has been developing with the connected devices: the *extimacy*. It can be defined by the choice to show a part of one's intimacy publicly on the social network. Tisseron suggests that the recourse to extimacy aims at reintegrating some elements exposed to others and validated by them. This "enacted" means could foster the regulation of the ideal instances: from the omnipotent ideals to the installation of self-confidence anchored in reality testing. Here, the metapsychological status of the projection-introjection and the identifications processes could be questioned. The social state of any individual subject has ever vowed him to the bodily interaction with the external objects in order to build his/her inner world (the maternal "capacity of reverie", the mirroring function, etc.) Jacques Lacan had already theorised the "extimacy" as the extension of the "intimate externality" in the process of sublimation, where the subjectivity and the symbolic order meet, in an aesthesic, aesthetic, ethical knotting. Even if Tisseron's conception of extimacy is quite different, it assumes similarly the project to extend, even enrich the boundaries of intimacy (Côté, 2011).

However, the social dimension seems rather different in the social network, since intimate and public spaces are melted and reconsidered; and since the realm of images prevails. The "virtual world" offers to the young generations ("Y" or "millenials", and "Z" generations) a quality of reality that still belongs to the "Real order". This reality can express in various dimensions: either a potential, or an actual, or a non-bodily one (non-tangible) (Tisseron, 2007. Indeed, the images born from the so-called "virtual world", once they have emerged from the invisible digital binary process of calculations, become visible and access to the materiality of the physics laws, stand to an analogical logic which leads to the representational system we're familiar with (Sultan, 2004). Besides, fantasies, structures of myths and symbolic language have something to do with the collective superego. The monsters here or there could still be coming from the most unknown territories of the mind and belonging to our collective ancestral Myths.

At a certain distance from the tangible reality (reality testing) of experiences and encounters, close to the Imaginary order (Lacan), the child or the adolescent finds in the computer world a new kind of contact with the other and with reality. The major concern would deal with the connection between the fantasy and the actualisation conducting to a possible sublimation, instead of discharge and acting. This arises the issue of the *locus* where the potential wishes can find an illusionary place before any realisation and that might open to a metaphoric meaning and language. Between creativity and negativity, the locus could be a "non-place" where new experiences can arise from the void, or an "anti-place" that hinders any play, any displacement, any transitional space and symbolisation, like a foreclosure.

We're indeed meeting several tracks to think about this new mind revolution. In a perspective full of hope where creativity still lies on a conception that takes into account postponement in the waiting of actualisation, the connective practices could foster the "representability" (Botella, S. and C., 2001) which promotes the first form of thinking based on the hallucinatory satisfaction. Differing, postponing, taking time for the not yet digestible psychic elements to meet reality could be compared to the preconception in waiting for the realisation (Bion). The model of the child's play (Winnicott) is valuable here again. To act "as if" before to be in contact and act "for real" might allow reality testing to be kept at the border and the data's flow to be kept in stock for a potential metabolisation. The network offers many opportunities for a different time to act and react: time for reflections, modifications on words or images, testing the good formulations before writing and showing to the others, time to listen to podcasts or recorded messages. But the capacity to differ, which leads to and sustains symbolisation and thoughts, might occur only on condition that the user possesses a capacity of judgement (for attribution and existence—Freud, 1925) and what Sophie Jehel (2018) calls a "posture of autonomy", rather than adhesive logics. The place of images in the digital logic might particularly illustrate the dilemma set in between the "mirroring function" (Freud, Winnicott) and the "bidimensionality" (Meltzer, 1980). We know since the pandemic that the meeting with a digital vision-image offers a kind of bodily "presence" that can give shape to a reflective, a specular encounter with a voice and a look that might contain and delineate the relation in an intimate space. Yet the screen vision fosters dissociation and dismantling, belongs to the part-object register, and contribute to unify the Self (such as the "a objects" defined by Lacan) if a skin-envelop is provided by the "consensuality" (Meltzer, 1980). On the surface, the psychic projections of two bodies emanating from the ego of each and potentially reflecting to one another (Freud, 1923) might convene the consistency and thickness of an inner space. On condition a "tridimentionality" has unfurled (Meltzer, 1980), the "3D" (even 4D) of a complete internalised "somato-psychic" universe, with its inner objects.

According to Meltzer, the private space "should not be revealed to the others in a dazzling way, in order not to disturb or depress them" (Meltzer, 1988). Lost in confusion, the superficial image of one's own not differentiated from the other, is stressed by the perverted ideal of "transparence". When everyone in the social network is invited to make and retouch his "extimate" image, the real otherness with its strange differences cannot really be found in the realm of the ego ideals. The searching for the self-containment/handling, the subjective "feeling of being", or the group's acknowledgment in the mirroring of the others' look might be a decoy, bringing its part of death and destruction; a perverted secretiveness hides beyond transparence.

Indeed, cybercrime and digital violence is now a serious subject matter that affects intimacy on several levels (legal, social, psychic...) The algorithms show a real postmodern figure of social evil in regard to the ideologies of consumerism and liberalism. Most of all, it arises the highest paranoid anxieties when the new persecutors are connected to anyone's intimate (extimate) room: a whole social group organisation personified by international political and economical actors, or unidentified malevolent individuals. Plots and spies, gangs and criminals do not only belong to the two discriminated registers that are either our fantasy, or the external reality, since the digital crime and its tracking spread out and infiltrate the connective intimacy. When many malevolent abusive acts are committed by adults on children and teenagers' extimate space (networks, games), when "revenge porn" and bullying are not controllable in the cyberspace, when the competitive quest for new consumers is dragging one's intimate wish to colonise it, we can hardly deny the "cyber-threat"; that of a traumatic external-internal agent intruding new kinds of intimate borders. We must assume that the collusion with the destructive and hostile fantasies is all the more disruptive and injuring that the child or the teenager feels as if he/she is standing inside his/her intimate private safe borders. Jehel defines the "adhesive posture" by the systematic tendency to "click" (acceptance of every solicitation from the web). This posture surely sticks to an archaic pattern referring to undifferentiation, symbiosis on its parasitic side (Bion, 1970), and the realm of the oceanic feeling in its lack of limits. We could also think that a perverse organisation takes place and submits the pseudo genuine intimacy to its control.

The outsider as a perverted non-bodily figure in the Oedipus pattern, versus the tricky figure of the polytropos Ulysses

Klein pictured five characters in the structure of the primal scene, according to the fantasy built by the infantile polymorphism: the mother and father, boy and girl, and the baby. Meltzer (1972) added what defines the perverse element, which tries to enter violently in the polymorphic family pattern: the "outsider" is pushed by envy and greed towards the unbearable beauty of the aesthetic object containing this scene. On the borders, an intrusive perverse pseudo-other is trying to colonise and degrade the beauty of the aesthetic intimate space.

This phantasmatic pattern, affected by splitting during childhood, is displaced during adolescence on the social groups that can contain and gather the split parts of the Self. The ideology of the social group can be that of a "gang", characterised by rebellion and seeking for the reproduction of the "secret and exciting investigation in the adulthood mystic". The function of the group is now partly dedicated to the connective group, whose members might sometimes not be embodied. Might this contact without the full bodily characteristics secrete a false kind of intimacy bound to an "extimate outsider", that could hinder the subjective construction? Then the extra-territorial status of intimacy would seem like a defensive maneuver against the painful shift of the boundaries and acceptance of the loss of the object. Schizo-paranoïde and perverse defences prevail under the appearances of smoke and mirrors of the digital screens. It might be all the more delicate to unveil this false dimension that the verbal and graphic communications look like symbolic and metaphoric language. Our infantile monsters can be worked through in the dream-work, are shaped in words representation in the narratives of the dream-telling. Perhaps an equivalence could be found through the medium of the visual representations presented on the website (gaming), if the frame offers a sufficient enough "malleable" quality (Milner, 1955). But the "representability" grounded in the preconscious takes shape through the cathexis of the *link* between affects and words weaving the bodily preverbal to the verbal language, producing the "talking effect" (Freud and Lacan) that addresses to an *embodied* Other.

In 1923 Freud proposed a new version of the Oedipal complex, built on the primal scene (Urszene) and the psychic bisexuality. This pattern settles the child as excluded from the "violent enough" parental intercourse, which enigmatic quality arises his curiosity. A contemporary fantasy of the origins might be nowadays reversing in a new version, according to which the parental couple is left aside and intrigued by their enigmatic child controlling the cyberspace and its intimate new spaces. We thus can recognise the triumph of the infantile omnipotence and its dreams of self-sufficiency—to which the Infantile (Guignard, 1996) of any adults can be submitted. However, on its fruitful side, this reversal of the Oedipal paradigm might also illustrate the multi-dimensions in which creativity is carried out by children and adolescents. As the mythic Ulysses (an adolescent figure) took the length of an Odyssey to recover the way back, edifying/conquering one's subjectivity involves creating other psychic territories of one's own with their singular frontiers, on the previous background: neither the same place, nor a strange unfamiliar one. The *kairos* (the appropriate temporality) of this journey-odyssey requires the *metis* (the cunning and trick) of Ulysses, a hero in search for his origins also called *polytropos*: the one who possesses many creative tricks.

A *"non-exclusive"* intimacy

The multiple realities disclosed by the means of new technologies and handled by children and teenagers reflect/echo in the actual issues about sexuality and gender, new procreations and parenthoods. The paradigms of intercrossing ("intersectionality") and complexity (Morin, 1990) to which Leticia Glocer-Fiorini (2007, 2019) refers about the feminine and the masculine, the maternal and the paternal, infuses the world of the youngest. When one exposes one's intimacy to more than a single one; when the mark of shared intimacy can exceed the number of two people; when gender identities does not stick to a choice between the one or the other; when sexuality spreads to various objects and realisations; when procreation and parenthood extend to multiple configurations; we should obviously infer that another pattern of human identifications and interactions shows up. This could be a major worry when the new modes of procreation and parenthood provide a circular Oedipus configuration rather than a triangular one (Guignard, 2019). But this real threat must not debar us from reviewing our theories. The binary logic that prevails in the occidental culture, hence the psychoanalytic field, calls for a deconstruction (Derrida, 1967), a semiotic analysis meant to reveal the journeys and *apories* in the discourses, and to maintain them in the "undecidable". If the theory of castration, according to Julio Moreno (2019), is a defensive theory that "hides the enigma of the difference of the sexes", the enigma might differ in different types of discourses that can coexist, rather than exclude one another. We must not exclude the alternatives of a non-exclusive conception of intimacy as a *discourse*. On condition that exclusion as a *fantasy* remains a structural element of the triangulation, which allows intimacy, and consequently the meaning of otherness and alterity.

"Non-exclusivity" can actually also be considered as a way out from the dyad to the third (- and more) object. Could we not then assume that exploring the "multiple" potentialities of the intimate spaces is for children and teenagers, an attempt to anchor to/find other symbolic meanings that could replace the lost emblems of a third party?

However, the symbolisation that promotes the metaphoric verbal language happens through bodily, sensori-motor experiences that are not social or cultural "conventions", but genuinely the creations of a dyad, held by drives and sexuality grounded on a biological soma and patterns. The encounter with the primary maternal space has created the conditions for an intimate psychic space; the primary feminine space opens to the intimacy of an erotic couple that contains the field of desire for the third (the Other's object). If this private intimate place is cathexed by the epistemophilic drives, if the renunciation of omnipotence and if loss of the depressive central position (Klein) are tolerable, then an integrated bisexuality based on the "symbolic character of difference" (Glocer-Fiorini, 2019), might lead the new generations to an *expanded* desire to explore and create an aesthetic intimate relationship with new other objects that include "others of the Other". Otherwise, multiplicity looks only like a hyperbolic version of the minute-splitting of schizo-paranoïd anxiety fighting against the shifts and losses inherent to the depressive position.

III The analyst facing the new intimacy of children and adolescents

Intimacy as the essence of the psyche is the space and the aim of psychoanalysis. The aesthetic encounter with the unknown makes the daily task of the analyst, observer and interpret of the psychic functioning of his patients belonging to a social-cultural context. Since the pandemic, lots of questions related to the modes of communication linked to the intimate spaces have been jumping into our faces. Until then, they were, for most of the psychoanalysts, stabbed by denial, resistance or reluctance, rejected in favour of the comfort of an established knowledge. If more than ever the uncertainty about the future does not allow any answer, we have to try to think the questions. Giving up a kind of certainty and open to an overwhelming "other-world" is all the more difficult that we might be less accustomed to what children and adolescents have already introjected or incorporated: a world based on connective logic, distant ties, deconstructed models of kinship and gender identities, severed from sexuality.

Elliott and Sarah: two short clinical examples of alter-natives

The "alter-natives" (children and teenagers) with another logic of the mind deserve more than ever our respect and delicacy towards their undecipherable private spaces, if we wish to communicate with them, learn from them and expand our knowledge. The psychoanalytic fields of childhood and adolescence seem to extend their spectrum from the peri-natal register to the late adulthood, following the cultural deconstruction of delineated states and genetic categories. These two vignettes illustrates how new elements appear in our daily clinic that force us to question the impact of a new social-cultural reality on the subjective psychic growth, and the ethical way for us to welcome it.

Elliot, ten years old, suffered from bullying, persistent obsessive thoughts and secondary encopresia when he began his treatment with me. His parents were worried by a call from the school alerting them about Elliott's despair. It was told to me that his bursting out angers were often calming down when he was watching a movie on TV being a little child, then with his switch game at six year old and later on (nine) when he was allowed to play on line (gaming). His intimate life became progressively filled with "virtual" activities, especially gaming with one friend, as a counter-point of an unbearable passivity with his peers that excluded him. But as the sophistication of the games increased, the playing put the two adversaries in fights that could not be overcome on the metaphoric level of the play. The distant partner of gaming turned to be a extremely sadistic persecutor, an extimate outsider who was crossing the fragile boundaries that were established between an inner world excessively controlled, invaded with split anal destructive objects, and an external threatening reality cathexed in a phobic way. Then the school called the parents because Elliot had threatened to commit a suicidal attempt at school. This new extimate space built in the distant exchange of the game obviously had appeared to be a defensive frontier, an "extended psychic space" (Jeammet) where the external objects of the external reality constituted a concrete support for his unbearable internal objects and fantasies. But the precarious boundaries had collapsed, revealing the despair underneath, the power of the destructive drives, the lack of a solid psychic intimacy. The medium of the game, virtually shared with a known schoolchild had the hybrid quality of a neither internal nor external territory whose boundaries could endlessly reverse into their opposite, impermeable to meaning and symbolisation.

During the session with Elliot, the only way to reach him was to enter his virtual world. Any other subject matter seemed flat and bi-dimensional, deprived of lively qualities and symbolic depth, like "symbolic equations" (Segall). I had to stand carefully on the borders, trying to understand and share the language of gaming, so as to try not to repeat the perverse intrusion of the outsider and be able to take progressively the place of transformative object (Bollas). On the other hand, I listened to the whole material as made of an inner fabric, inhabited with split parts and objects actively circulating through projective identifications. The extimate experience happening in the external world shared the same destiny *in my mind* as the expression of his fantasies. But I was wondering if I could really understand the extended impact of his gaming world and negotiate with these new patterns of exchanges. Following Elliot step by step, I had to contain his anxieties aroused by a threatening intimacy coming from outside and inside without discrimination. Being able to welcome my feeling of strangeness and disorientation towards an ambiguous extra-territory, was the first move towards the hope to co-construct an aesthetic experience in a safe protected extra-territorial zone.

Sarah was seduced by an older woman (30 years of age) on the social network at 14. She could realise the traumatic quality of the event when she began a therapy with me, aged 19. The connective sexualised relationship with the woman that had lasted several years, seemed to have acquired the psychic status of a "bizarre object" (Bion), an obtrusive inner outsider on which it was very difficult to think and talk about during the sessions. Neither could she have a consistent narrative about her mother. But she could easily mention her relationship with her actual girlfriend who had "saved" her from intimate seclusion, constant feelings of despair and hysteric symptoms, after her relationship with the feminine rapist ended. Her girlfriend was cathexed as an idealised undifferentiated part of herself, a saver maternal part-object split from the combined parents in which a masculine/paternal part-object much devaluated concealed the damaged primal object. We were wandering together within the boundaries of her representative landscape of sexual identifications. A shape in my mind was progressively delineating for her homosexual cathexis. But during one session, Sarah talked about the tension occurring in her couple because her girlfriend was not feeling well for some times and was too much demanding for support, since she had now adopted the non-binary gender. Then the "she" (the girlfriend) suddenly became a "he" in the discourse of Sarah. While my previous representation of the girlfriend was collapsing in a hazy shade of thoughts, I felt the boundaries of my own identity vacillating for a while. I did not know any more what I had heard and experienced before with this patient. This short moment of blank thought was followed by the feeling of being forced not to have the visual image of a girl, and not to utter any feminine words. I could only say to Sarah how difficult and strange it might be to have to change abruptly the way of naming and thinking about her girlfriend, who was now becoming a boyfriend, as I was experiencing it now with her.

This example illustrates some arising questions about our conceptual tools to the test of the new clinical configurations of the gender issues. Since the psychic material is born in the session and in the analytical field (Baranger M. and W.), how can we work it through and part the elements belonging to the external reality from the psychic dynamic ones—some of which I contributed to, as a member of the analytic couple? It was my first clinical contact with the question of gender identity. Having afterwards experienced many of these situations with young patients without the same intense feeling of confusion and derealisation, should I not assume that getting more acquainted to a new cultural paradigm changes the frame (borders) of my perception?

I had assumed that my counter-transference feelings carried out by projective identifications brought me close to Sarah's psychic movements. As I had experienced it during the session, her girlfriend had became an uncanny, rejected object—when her gender status had reversed as well as her function (saver/persecutor-victim)—reproducing the traumatic impingement of the first event with the older woman. Alike this first event with the woman on the social network, the bodily reality was stabbed by disavowal. It had no place to anchor the concreteness of the con-sensual body in an embodied relation. But the bodily print in the transference also contained the potentiality of a dangerous seductive intimacy. Could this usual pervasive effect of the analytic meeting have increased because of a non-qualification (non-binary) of a stranger body for us both? Could this uncanny experience during the session be *only* related to the dimension of the threatening acceptance of bisexuality for Sarah?

The risk of a "traumatogenic" counter-transference

According to Meltzer (1967), the transference deserves a long development of the analytical process for the analyst to grasp the aesthetic modalities of thoughts created by the analysis and its method. When defences against the aesthetic impact or *traumatic events* hinder the sensibility to beauty, the analytic work might be embroiled in the crucial need to "find again the aesthetic object" and lead to catastrophic psychosomatic reactions. But the traumatic might as well locate in the analytic field, especially in the way the psychoanalyst handles the transference and responds to it.

Referring to Ferenczi, Thierry Bokanowski (2001) recalls that the "trauma" (the negative action of the economic overflow on the psychic organisation) is leading to archaic and primitive defences of the nascent ego (such as splitting-and-idealisation, denial, pathological projective identification…) and creating "blank psychic zones" of unrepresented elements. How can we measure the traumatic impact on our psyches, of the huge epistemological shift carried out by our little and teenage patients? It seems that reality goes faster than our capability to think it. Lost in a very unknown zone, we might be struck by the traumatic effect of a new kind of uncanny, not yet thinkable. Among the psychic elements emerging from a new connective sensibility (aesthesis) of our young patients, we might not be able to distinguish. Some might belong to an inner intimate world of supple identifications and discriminated objects; others belong either to an enclosed system with rigid and obtrusive objects that have been incorporated in a melancholic way such as "crypts" (Torok N. and M.), or to a hyper-projective and unsafe space unable to contain and produce intimate aesthetic objects. There, the "transformation in hallucinosis" and the "hyperbolic projection" (Bion) prevail. To be able to metabolise the beta-elements (Bion) thanks to an alpha-function (the maternal capacity of reverie) requires a non-iatrogenic psychic apparatus. When facing the sensorial, somatic unknown beta-elements of our patients, especially with children and teenagers, we know as analysts that we run many dangers, mostly of projective and narcissistic essence. The risk, with our skilled and enigmatic young patients, stresses the epistemological gap that keeps us at a far distance.

There might be two extremities on the scale of the technical risks dragged by our counter-transference. On the one hand, our ignorance might push us to intrude violently their mind so as to possess their skill and knowledge, reproducing the abusive "confusion of tongues" between the child and the seductive adult (Ferenczi). In this altered version, our own envy towards the enigma of their special otherness can induce a kind of reversal: we would be the ones subjected to their unknown enigmatic tongue. Our own Infantile then leads the movement in the transference. On the other hand, we might fill and force their psyche with old reassuring and saturated theories (such as "stopper interpretations" and "blind spots", Guignard, 1996).

The Infantile: a reliable concept of psychoanalysis

The psychoanalytical community has begun to question its concepts, such as the feminine, which we can no longer consider as a strong bedrock articulated to the phallic order. If the Oedipus organisation remains a cornerstone of our theory, its relevance does not seem to reside in a structural complex any more. However, in a society where paradoxes and primary defences prevail, the infantile sexuality could still provide the invariants that "resist"—as Guignard formulates it. Our epistemological task is to conceive bonds and bridges *in-between* what stands as a human psychic and somatic invariant, and the shifting elements that are yet necessary to generate the infantile bisexuality. Such positioning takes into account the "regredient" movement of the psychoanalytical *epistémé* confronted by the contemporary clinic of the borders. As Green drew attention to (1990), the Freudian conception of the borders between neurosis and psychosis in his latest works (Freud, 1924, 1937) called for an opening to the factors of *transition*, altogether with the necessary and moveable splits. In the developmental process, the passages from one territory of the mind to another are much more numerous than the delineated and contrasted states. Following the Freudian proposals, passages and transitions could be considered as the locus of *in-between bonds*—also shaped like a "gap" (Jullien, 2012)—that give a space in which the "nothing-yet" resides and where the difference, the unknown can occur. As Derrida writes it, the "*differance*" (what differs) makes a step aside and overtakes the binary dialectical opposition to open to a work of unknown thoughts-to-come. When Bion conceptualised the relation container-content with the feminine-masculine symbols, it conveyed the model of a psychic intimate space where the parental intercourse can take place and give birth to a *third place* of creation. The intimacy of this erotic union requires a bond (the link "-") that assumes metaphorically the "meta-" dimension (transformation and abstraction) created by the relation between, at least, two elements. The passage from one element to another is offering an "interstitial" space where the traffic of different elements generates an enigmatic *differance*.

In the same perspective, Guignard conceived the Infantile as a "third concept" (2014). This conception goes a little further than the "third-party" psychoanalytical concept, since it contains but exceeds the idea of separation and loss towards creation (poïesis), to promote the *in-between* notion. The "third concept" provides a meta- concept to contain the "transformative interaction of the psychic transmitters" and refers to Bion's model of cesura considering the *function of the bond* between two elements in a dynamic oscillation, after Freud's pattern of synaptic psychic transmission (1895) and Klein's projective identification. As conceptualised by Guignard, the Infantile is a sensible dynamic space that gathers the archaic and primary sensori-motor experiences. It conveys the protosymbolic shapes for any emotional experience to happen all life long. In a metaphoric meaning, it promotes the seesaw movements back and forth between the different libidinal organisations, the different metapsychological instances and topics, as the crucible of fantasies, psychic transformations and the operator leading to the symbolic operations. The concept of the Infantile standing as the new bedrock for our theories either to emerge or to sink remains a strong counterpoint to the realm of the "Real". Children and adolescent stand, as equilibrists, *in-between* several new extended or shortened borders, unfolding an extra-territorial subjectivity and prob-ably showing us the way to resist and to adjust to the Real. The extra-territoriality as a new production of the Infantile could open potential third spaces, with their promises, their risks and dead-ends.

Conclusion

Obviously, the shifting boundaries of intimate spaces during childhood and adolescence echoes the worldwide changes that affect us all. Thanks to our little patients and teenagers, we will be able to witness the impact of the Real order (Lacan) on the psychic construction of subjectivity, even if our own psychic tools are too limited to be aware of the long-term effects. In favour of the reality principle, these two main infantile shapes will still be challenging the painful discovery of a "loss in progress" that constitutes *the nucleus* of human destiny. However, we should perhaps back up with the concept of "reliance" (Kristeva, 2019), a maternal "urgent state of life" in which Eros gathers the living substance, preserves it and spreads the libidinal drive into the tender tide: an ethos for a shared humanity. As Morin (2020) recently wrote, "Let's change of way" to turn toward a politics of humanity. Seeking for human unity and collective singularities appears to be the watchword of the young generations. With no wonder, this meets the labour of psychoanalysis: to differentiate among the instances, the inner objects, the inside and the outside, in order to integrate every single entity within a unified Self.

Notes

1 Guignard has conceived this hypothesis for some time now (1984, 1989).
2 For instance, the IEMP (Institute for the Medical and Preventive Education), a public organisation sustained by the national Health Department, counts emi-nent scientific members that published in 2018 a campaign on "The good use of digital screens" (www.institut-iemp.com).
3 Lecture at the Collège de France: "Where does computer science go?" (4 March 2019).

References

Abraham, N.and Torok, M. 1978/1987. *L'Ecorce et le noyau*. Paris: Flammarion.

Anzieu, D. 1974/1997. *Le Moi-peau*. Paris: Dunod.

Baranger, M.and W. 1961. La situation analytique comme champ dynamique(trans. Fr. L. de Urtebey), *Rev Fr Psychan.*, 49(6): 1543–1572.

Bick E. 1967/2007. L'expérience de la peau dans les relations d'objets précoces. In Meg Harris William (dir.). *Les écrits de Martha Harris et d'Esther Bick*. Larmor-Plage: Editions du Hublot, 135–139.

Bion, W.R. 1962/1984. *Learning from experience*. London: Routledge.

Bion, W.R. 1965/2002. *Transformations. Passage de l'apprentissage à la croissance*. Paris: Puf.

Bion, W.R. 1970/1984. *Attention and Interpretation*. London: Routledge.

Bokanowski, T. 2002. Traumatisme, traumatique, trauma, *Rev Fr Psychanal*, 66(3): 745–757.

Bollas, C. 1989. L'objet transformationnel, *Rev Fr Psychan.*, 53(4): 1181–1199.

Bronner, G. 2021. *Apocalypse cognitive*. Paris, Puf.

Botella, C. et S. 2001/2007. *La Figurabilité psychique*. Paris: In Press.

Côté, J.F. 2011. Des origines artistiques de l'extimité à une esthétique généralisée des démocraties de masse chez Andy Warhol, *Le Texte étranger*, 8. Online: www. univ-paris8.fr/dela/etranger/pages/8/cote.html.

Derrida, J. (1967/2003), Freud et la scène de l'écriture, in *L'écriture et la différence*. Paris: Le Seuil.

Derrida, J. 1972/1989. La Pharmacie de Platon. In Platon, *Phèdre*. Paris: Flammarion.

Ferenczi S., 1931/1982. Analyse d'enfants avec des adultes. In *Œuvres complètes IV, 1927-1933*. Paris: Payot, 98–112.

Ferenczi, S., 1932/1982. Confusion des langues entre les adultes et les enfants. In *Œuvres complètes IV, 1927-1933*. Paris: Payot, 125–138.

Freud, S. 1895/2006. Projet d'une psychologie. *Lettres à Wilhem Fliess: 1887–1904*. Paris: Puf, 593–693.

Freud, S. 1915/1968. *Pulsions et destins des pulsions*. In: *Métapsychologie*. Paris: Gallimard.

Freud, S. 1923/1981. Le Moi et le ça. In: *Essais de psychanalyse*. Paris: Payot.

Freud, S. 1925/1985. La Négation. In: *Résultats, Idées, Problèmes II*. Paris: Puf.

Glocer-Fiorini, L. 2007. *Deconstructing the feminine. Psychoanalysis, Gender and Theory of complexity*. London: Karnac.

Glocer-Fiorini, L. 2019. The maternal and the paternal in the 21st century. Shifting territories, Panel on The feminine, the maternal, the masculine, the paternal, in today's parenthood. IPA Congress on *The Feminine*, London, 27 July 2019.

Green, A. 1990. *La Folie privée. Psychanalyse des cas-limites*. Paris: Gallimard.

Guignard, F. 1996. *Au vif de l'Infantile*. Lausanne: delachaux et niestlé.

Guignard, F. 2014. Quels concepts métapsychologiques pour le clinique aujourd'-hui? Les concepts de troisième type. In: Passone, S.M. and Guignard, F., *Psychanalyse de l'enfant et de l'adolescent. Etats des lieux et perspectives*. Paris: In Press.

Guignard, F. 2019. The Maternal and the Feminine: two primal aeras of psychic development, object relations and identifications. Présentation IPA Pre-congress, London 24 July 2019.

Guignard, F. 2019. Oedipus blown up and the Infantile omniprésent. Présentation IPA Congress on *The Feminine*, London, 27 July 2019.

Gutton, P. 1997. Découvrir le pubertaire, *Adolescence, special edition, 2001*:9–14.

Gutton, P. 2004. La Virtualité et ses conduites, *Adolescence*, 47, Paris: GREUPP.

Gutton, P. 2013. *Le Pubertaire*. Paris: Puf.

Jehel, S. 2018. Les adolescents face aux violences numériques, *Terminal 123⊠2018*. DOI: https://doi.org/10.4000/terminal.3226.

Jullien, F. 2012. *L'écart et l'entre. Leçon inaugurale de la chaire sur l'altérité*. Paris: Galilée.

Kahn, M. 1983. *Hidden Selves, Between Theory and Practice in Psychoanalysis*. London: The Hogarth Press and Institute of Psycho-analysis.

Kelly-Lainé, K. 2017. Langage, exil et identité intime: la dynamique inconsciente de l'enfance perdue, *Bull Féd Eur Psychanal*, 71: 188–198.

Kristeva, J. 2011. La reliance, ou de l'érotisme maternel, *Rev Fr Psychan*, 75(5): 1559–1570.

Lemma, A. 2015. Psychoanalysis in the times of technoculture: Some reflections on the fate of the body in virtual space, *Int J Psychoanal*, 96: 569–582.

Meltzer, D. 1972/1977. *Les structures sexuelles de la vie psychique*. Paris: Payot.

Meltzer, D., Bremner, J., Hoxter, S., Weddel, D., Wittenberg, I. and Haag, G. 1980. *Explorations dans le monde de l'autisme. Etude psychanalytique*. Paris: Payot.

Meltzer, D. 1987/2013. Présence de l'objet et séparation d'avec lui. Attaques envieuses et intolérance du conflit esthétique. In: *Donald Meltzer à Paris, conférences et séminaires au GERPEN* (dir. J. Touzé). Larmor Page: Editions du Hublot.

Meltzer, D. 1988/2000. *L'appréhension de la beauté*. Larmor-Plage: Editions du Hublot.

Milner, M. 1955/2004. The role of illusion in the formation of symbol. In: *Psychoanalysis and art, Kleinien perspectives*. London: Routledge.

Moreno, J. 2019. "Is it there a feminine/masculine struggle or just a difference?", Panel on The feminine, the maternal, the masculine, the paternal, in today's parenthood, IPA Congress on *The Feminine*, London, 27 July2019.

Moreno, J. 2018. "The origin of humans", EPF 31th Annual Conference, *The origin of life*, Warsaw, March.

Morin, E. 1990. *Introduction à la pensée complexe*. Paris: Le Seuil.

Morin, E. 2020. *Changeons de voie*. Paris: Denoël.

Naccache, L. 2020. *Le cinema intérieur, Projection privée au coeur de la conscience*. Paris: Odile Jacob.

Segal, H. 1957/1979. Post-scriptum. Notes sur la formation des symboles. In *Délires et créativité. Essais de psychanalyse clinique et théorique*. Paris: Editions des femmes, 112–120.

Sultan, J. 2004. L'image virtuelle n'existe pas, Construction d'un imaginaire, *Adolescence*, 47: 33–42.

Tisseron, S. 2007. De l'intimité librement exposée à l'intimité menacée, in VST—Vie sociale et traitements, *Revue des CEMEA*, 93(1): 74–76. Online: www.cairn.info/revue-vie-sociale-et-traitements-2007-1-page-74.htm.

Tisseron, S. 2011. Intimité et extimité, *Communications*, 2011/1 (no. 88), 83–91.

Winnicott, D. 1975/1986. *Jeu et Réalité, L'espace potentiel*. Paris: Gallimard.

3 The Oblivious Object

Mary T. Brady, PhD

This chapter will consider children with an unconscious relation to an "oblivious object". I have spent time considering these issues because they pertain to children (or adults) who tend to find the analyst useless. The conceptualisation of an unconscious relationship to a "stupid object" was introduced by Alvarez (2012). Her 2012 chapter discusses narcissism, or what presents like narcissism in children (children whom she aptly describes as "not easy to like"). The conceptualisation of children with an unconscious relation to an "oblivious object",[1] is related and presents additional challenges for clinicians to identify and to work with. Such children might admire their sometimes highly accomplished parents, yet unconsciously experience their object(s) as oblivious to their internal world. The parents I am describing are well in certain respects, but chronically unavailable to complex or messy emotions in their children. Conceptualisations of unconscious relationships to stupid or oblivious objects are, of course, relevant in adults as well. But here, I discuss these issues in children as it can be informative to see troubling object relations early in their development.

I will first describe Alvarez's description of a stupid object and some of her ideas regarding narcissism in children. I will then briefly relate Klein's and Bion's theories of unconscious object relations, as underpinnings for the consideration of a stupid or an oblivious object. I will next differentiate an "oblivious" from a "stupid" object, although such conceptualisations are closely related. I will then provide clinical material of a thirteen-year-old girl in treatment, in order to consider these ideas. I will also describe the somewhat normal developmental tendency for adolescents to consider adults as oblivious.

The Stupid Object[2]

Alvarez has described a type of internal object, which is not exactly felt to be bad, but rather stupid and useless. She observed this unconscious object relation in some children of drug addicts, alcoholics, or in cases of maternal depression. Such children lay parent dolls on the floor when

DOI: 10.4324/9781003246749-3

using the doll house—literally reflecting a sense of no figure to look up to. Alvarez comments that the lack of someone to look up to can lead to cognitive dullness in a child as there is no magnet, no mystery, and insufficient excitement to evoke any curiosity. Such children have no concept of an object who is intelligent—no sense of an adult having an interested and interesting mind. These children see their internal object and potentially adults in general as weak, useless, unprotective and unprotected.

Alvarez's description of "stupid" objects overlaps with depressed or damaged objects. It might be possible for children to see the limitations in such objects and gradually differentiate them from other adults. When problems in parents (such as drug addiction, alcoholism or depression) are named in the environment it is easier for children to make differentiations. For instance, I treated a boy from a wealthy family whose mother suffered from depression. His memories of her from his early childhood are all of her being in bed. While he loved her, he certainly saw her as useless. He saw his multiple nannies and other household staff as more emotionally and practically available, but he was never really their primary concern. His sense of his mother's limitations (which of course she did not want to suffer), were not denied in the family and could be named. He experienced the depressed aspect of his mother as uninterested, and so in Alvarez's terms "stupid"—not capable of expressing interest in him, nor generating interest from him. As Alvarez says, children of such parents do not see the parent as bad, but as useless. We could wonder if a "bad" object could be more animating for a child (than a stupid object), in that the child might feel hate towards their parent instead of indifference. Of course, these distinctions are to aid our thinking and are not absolute. An absent enough object, (such as for the boy I am referring to), does also generate some hatred, albeit towards a weak/"stupid" object.

Alvarez suggests that for therapists, the experience of being with an emotionally deprived child with a stupid, uninteresting object might be similar to being with a devaluing child, in that the therapist might experience him/ herself as uninteresting. Such distinctions can meaningfully guide therapists in our reflections and interventions.

Alvarez describes subtypes of narcissistic states of mind in children. She differentiates normal self-centeredness from "pathological" self-centeredness in terms of the normal child's ability to acknowledge nurturing. Alvarez says that the sense of a stupid object might arise in a child with some beginning experience of a lively object, but who suffers a narcissistic injury. In Bionian terms, the unmetabolised experience of narcissistic injury is projected into the object—hopefully to occasion emotional work in the parent or analyst. If the narcissistic woundedness is not transformed, a child might develop a more ongoing reliance on contempt. Alvarez notes that a more complacent attitude of contempt can signal the beginning of a more permanent sense of superiority in a child.

Unconscious Object Relations

Alvarez uses Klein's conceptualisation of an internal world organised around central unconscious relationships between aspects of the self and complementary and corresponding objects (Klein, 1975). I am also placing this understanding of unconscious object relations within Bion's (1962) conceptualisation of container/contained.

The concept of an internal object is not intended to imply an exact representation of a parent, but to be influenced by aspects of the object, as well as phantasies of the object also affected by the child's own processes. For instance, an aspect of a parent at a particularly difficult time, might be internalised by a child and have outsize influence on the child. In addition, children relate to different facets of their object representation at different moments, for instance at periods of comparative ease or comparative strain.

Klein (1975) saw an infant's earliest development as characterised by primitive phantasies. In her view, the infant's experience of loving caretaking confirms the sense of a good phantasied object or softens the phantasy of a bad object. She saw the primary object of earliest development (the paranoid-schizoid phase) as experienced alternatively as ideal or persecutory, owing to splitting processes and paranoid anxiety. Splitting allows the infant to make order out of chaotic experience. A predominance of good over bad experiences is necessary in order to be able to proceed to the next stage, the depressive position. Klein did not view that development is based solely on the internalisation of good or bad experiences, but that an internal predisposition to envy might modify gratifying experiences.

Klein held that the badness or anxiety too difficult to experience inside the self is evacuated out into the other, through projective identification. Bion (1962) acknowledged Klein for her insights into projective identification, but also took the concept in an expansive, new direction. He saw projective identification as not just a mechanism of defence, but as the first mode of communication between mother and infant—as the first rudiment of thinking.

In Bion's view, the infant conveys his fears to his mother[3] by projecting them into her for her to receive and know. The mother hopefully receives the fears and struggles to contain them by giving them meaning. The child's gradual ability to know him or herself is facilitated by being taken in and known in his mother's mind. I consider this a territory where the sense of an "oblivious object" can develop. Some of the children I am considering have loving parents, but parents who have little idea what to do with a child's emotional experience. This leaves a divided experience for the child, conscious love and admiration for and from the parent(s), but with little hope for anything better than oblivious misattunement.

According to Bion, reverie is the capacity of the primary object to love and think about his or her infant, gradually allowing the infant to internalise a parent who is able to think. The infant can ideally absorb the experience that his or her feelings can be modified, understood and related to. The lack of the experience of reverie leaves the infant without the sense that emotional experiences can be thought about. Sometimes, "oblivious" parents have some recognition that they do not understand their child (this was the case for the mother of Frances, whom I will describe below). Such parents do not know what to do with emotion, but rather turn to other aspects of themselves or their child—such as an emphasis on academic or athletic success. Some parents avoid any knowledge of their lack of emotional understanding of their children and emphasise their material provision for the child.

Bion saw the personality as constituted by two elements—contained and container—in a dynamic relationship, with the contained continually seeking a container. In an attuned relationship between a mother and baby, a sense of a loving relationship can be internalised into the infant's personality, which transforms into an internal healthy container and contained dynamic in the infant. Alternatively, in a misattuned relationship between a mother and baby, a useless container can be internalised—for example, an obliviousness to one's own experiences. In Bionian terms, oblivious containment creates starved emotional contents, as well as oblivious internal containment.

The analyst might need to be careful not to defensively reject the projective identification of obliviousness. Tolerating this projection can gradually lead to understanding the child's expectation of obliviousness. Paradoxically, it might be the analyst's willingness to be experienced as oblivious that can allow the child to gradually internalise an object who does not evade the child's experience. On the other hand, the child's disinterest in the analyst might need to be challenged for some sort of break-through to a new experience.

The Oblivious Object

Much has been written (e.g., Mondzrak, 2012) suggesting a contemporary culture of narcissism, abandoning children into narcissistic formations. Societal and parental overvaluation of success and undervaluation of children's inner worlds can be the context for the development of an "oblivious object". These children might see their parents as highly intelligent in the external world and even idealise and emulate them, but unconsciously experience their parents as unavailable to their deeper selves. Such parents either do not know what to do with their children's emotional experience or are actively avoidant of any difficult emotion in their children. Unfortunately, children might unconsciously identify with not just their parents' professional success, but also their emotional avoidance.

Another variant of this problem is parents who also idealise their children, in part to distance themselves from their children's emotional problems. At times parents seemingly generously interpret their children's actions as positive, when they are in fact something else. For instance, eighteen-year-old Stephen related a memory in which he had been embarrassed by his father questioning a waiter. His father noted how "kind" his son was to be concerned for the waiter. Children's discomfort with parents drawing attention to themselves is fairly common, especially at ages when the children themselves are particularly self-conscious. So, while a rather ordinary experience, Stephen was feeling critical of his father. Father's idealising of his son left no room for father to notice criticism and be strong enough to think about it. While Stephen's parents seem comparatively benign, their consistent idealisation of their son (including his academic excellence), ignored his multiple difficulties. This left him feeling both he and his parents were oblivious to any way to recognise and approach his problems. His underlying rage at his parents' obliviousness further separated him from them. Neither he nor they really understood his distance from them, but this distance cut him off from taking in the genuinely good qualities they had to offer. His alienation from them was part of the referring issue. I will give a vignette to convey how his sense of an oblivious or useless object came up in the treatment and how his relationship to an oblivious object also left him oblivious to others.

When S. started treatment, he refused regular meetings with me. I decided to go along with this for a time, to see if his need to come on his own terms might eventually yield to some deeper entry into the work. After some months I told him I would no longer work on this basis, and he was welcome to return, if he could see his way to meeting regularly. Several months later, he returned. Over the next year we met once, then twice weekly, but he missed many sessions without notice. We worked through some of the meanings of these withdrawals, including his fear of his suicidal thoughts and his fear he was mentally ill. Over the next year he increased from three to then four weekly sessions. He attended his sessions steadily.

In this context, we were in a period when Stephen mainly wanted me to let him talk uninterrupted in his sessions. During this particular session I was comfortable with this implicit arrangement, feeling he needed to play in the presence of an 'environmental mother' (Winnicott, 1959). I was interested in his various riffs throughout the session. As the session drew to an end, I commented, "I think you know I am with you even when I am silent". S. responded, "That doesn't seem important, what's important is what I'm talking about". At this point my heart dropped, as I felt I'd allowed him to play out a scene in which he is addicted to his self-importance and my irrelevance. I said, "You experience me as little more than a place holder. I think we have to deal with how disruptive it feels to you when someone else comes in". S. responded, "What do other people give me? I'm being honest. Well, I guess I've gotten laid three times. What do you want from me?"

Stephen was silent the first half of the next session. I then said, "I got impatient about you pushing me away last session and you felt attacked". S. responded, "Everyone sucks. What's wrong with being an angry person?" I said, "It isn't actually strong to just be aggressive". S. said, "There are a lot of things to be critical of. I don't feel much care". I responded, "You're getting too used to pushing people away and then you can't see what can happen with another person". I said, "You wind up living in a world of one". (He has subsequently come back to this comment several times.)

The next session Stephen started by reading a passage from a memoir in which the writer describes a psychiatrist's description of her during a breakdown as almost entirely alienated from other humans' feelings. I commented, "That's a scary picture". This period felt like a turning point in our work. I saw S. as unable to deal with my or others' positive or negative feelings toward him. His withdrawal seemed to imply a sense of himself at an emotional level as not having anything to offer (while being exceptional intellectually). His parents had been benign, but oblivious to how to deal with his difficult feeling. He had radically withdrawn from them. They were concerned about this withdrawal and initiated treatment because of it. However, they were oblivious as to how to step into his anger. Thus, obliviousness occurred at multiple levels here. His sense of an oblivious object created a rage in S., which he felt his object(s) were unable to deal with. Their unwillingness or inability to deal with his anger added to his contempt.

Stephen's assumption of my uselessness had to be confronted to begin to face his contempt, as well as the vast insecurity that underlay his endless criticism. I felt that to some degree I had to force my way in with S. He would have been content for some time to treat me as useless even though he was using me. His indifference or obliviousness to my experience was parallel to an unconscious parental communication of "we don't care how you feel as long as you continue to excel and don't disturb our emotional equilibrium".

I have written elsewhere (Brady, 2015) about a developmentally "normal" attitude adolescents have toward parents/adults as oblivious. Adolescents often accuse even seemingly attentive parents of being oblivious. I see the experience of obliviousness as a part of the adolescent separation process. Separation processes can leave adolescents feeling cut off both from their real external parents and also from their experience of an inner helpful object. Parents are pushed away and yet needed. Developmentally "normal" accusations of obliviousness can be exacerbated when there is some real way the parent is checked out or emotionally unavailable.

Next, I will examine the concept of an "oblivious object" in a 13-year-old girl of an educated and affluent family. This girl was quite consciously idealising of her successful and affectionate parents. Her sense of the obliviousness of her object needed to arise in our relationship and be understood in the transference-countertransference field. Such work might allow a beginning sense of an object who can be of emotional use to a child.

"Frances"

Frances was referred after she told her mother she felt very anxious and "not right in the head". She had told her mother tearfully: "I have a crushing in my head, and I shouldn't be alive".

F. attends a private school. Her parents described F. as, "good inter-personally—a reluctant leader who is curious and political". Her parents reported a history of depression on both sides of the family. Mother suffered panic attacks in her early twenties and tried therapy but said: "I didn't take to it. I tough things out".

Pregnancy and delivery were normal. F. was breast-fed. Mother went back to full-time work when F. was three months old. Mother told me that F., "refused to eat from the au pair the first week I went back to work". Father laughingly described this as F. being "stubborn". I commented: "This seemed far too young for stubbornness, but rather seemed a sign of distress". Mother said: "I did think F. was distressed and that, then as now, I would not work if F. needed me, but that I didn't know what to do". Compared with father, mother had some sense that her infant was emotionally distraught but was unable to use her perception to respond emotionally and practically.

Many near catastrophic difficulties preceded F.'s younger sister's birth, when F. was five. F. "was stand-offish" after her sister's birth. F.'s eight-year-old sister sleeps in the parents' bed. Mother started a demanding job a year prior to F. beginning treatment and travels for work intermittently. F. is anxious and has stomach aches when her mother is away.

Course of Treatment

My initial impression upon meeting F. was that she was in much worse psychological condition than her parents had conveyed. It felt eerie to be with her. She only spoke if I made a comment or asked a question. When F did speak, what she said was often gripping. In the first session F. told me she felt, "in a deep hole, with a shovel instead of a rope". She said in fourth and fifth grades she had felt, "not good, not bad, murky" and in sixth grade, "I felt doomed and unreal". She currently (summer before seventh grade) often feels like, "I am watching myself". I had the impression that she was having a dissociative experience of removal from herself. I inquired into her having told her parents, "I shouldn't be alive". She replied, " I don't want to kill myself; I just wish I could evaporate".

I felt concerned in early sessions that F. could be having a breakdown or entering into a major mental illness. I felt some hope when she came in to the second session and said, "I like your hair style". I tried to ask what she meant, but she could not elaborate. I took the comment as some bit of positive feeling towards me. She also said, "I dreamed I had a puppy with me that I held throughout the day". I said, "The puppy may be a part of yourself that you feel some willingness that we care for". She seemed to agree but could not say more. I told F.'s parents that she was significantly depressed and anxious and recommended that she begin a twice-weekly treatment.

F. had a planned two weeks away coming up, the first week a family vacation and the second week to a friend's country home, which she had visited before. I asked what it might feel like for us to have a break so soon after starting. She replied, "lonely, but you could send me a letter". I soon received an urgent message from mother that F. felt too anxious to go to her friend's house. Her parents agreed for her to stay home. When she came in, F. said, "I feel depressed and hopeless, like someone turned the lights off". I felt very concerned about F.'s state and suggested to her parents that I see her each day that week, which they agreed to. I told them, "She has hidden some of how bad she has been feeling because she feels she is supposed to perform".

F. said during that week, "I feel empty, I feel worse and worse until I blank out," and described "suffocating panic". She denied hallucinations or delusions. I said, "It is very important that your parents and I stay close to you when you are feeling like this". I mentioned the possibility of medication to F. and asked how she felt about it. She said, "I don't care". In a later session I told F., "Medication is no substitute for our feeling close and would not be forever, but it could help you feel better now". I said I was open to hearing whether what she was going through felt like too much for her. Soon after, F. told me that she did want to start medication. The psychiatrists I normally work with were away on vacation, so I sought out someone who could see her. The psychiatrist said F. had been having "panic like events" and intense fears with quasi-suicidal thoughts. He said her parents were concerned at the frequency I was seeing F. (three sessions a week at this point) and that he had agreed with them that it seemed excessive.

While F.'s parents had initially seemed reasonably trusting, their support wavered in this period. They expressed confusion as to how to know we were on the right track. I said I could understand their worry about whether I was giving their daughter the right care, but that it was a good sign that she was talking with me. Meanwhile, I dreamed I was on a ship turning upside down, which meant there would be water in every floor of the ship. There would be an air pocket on each floor, but I would be underwater for a time, while everything went upside down. My dream reflected my anxiety about F., but also the faltering support I had. I asked her parents to come in and meet with me to talk about this directly. I said, "When a child feels overwhelmed it is really important that the adults around them come together". Without an alliance it would be very hard to work in this situation. During this period, F. talked at length about a television show which depicts characters who are sucked into a strange, parallel universe.

Meanwhile F. started on an anti-depressant, which was clearly helpful. Her crushing, suffocating anxiety decreased.

The parents occasionally cancelled my appts. with F. I told them that F. needed to see that our appointments were being treated as important. Shortly after this I came out to the office to collect F. for an appointment. She was not there, but her mother was. She said F. was out in the car, not wanting to come in because she was upset about school and wanted to go home. I suggested to mother that I go down and speak with F. in the car. I told F. that it was especially important we be together when she was upset, so she could get more used to having emotions when she was with me. F. was able to come in and have the session. Mother had been able to support the treatment in not acceding to F.'s testing of the solidity of our work. Here, mother was able to not be oblivious to F.'s need for treatment and my need for mother's support. Since this crisis period our work has been more stable. F. is still silent unless I start us off. She then speaks in an animated manner. She does not like to talk about her anxiety because she feels it will start again.

At the time of the session I will provide, F. had just reduced to two sessions a week, five months into treatment. My current struggle centres on helping F. to deal with her difficulties when she is also genuinely feeling better.

F. is on time, slight smile to me as I get her in the Waiting Room. She picks up her folder of drawings and goes to sit cross-legged on the couch. She starts to colour in the shapes of the outlines she made last time. She is silent. I think about whether to let the silence extend. After a few minutes, I say:

A: I was thinking it feels like a ritual when you pick up the markers and start to draw. Like it almost would feel strange to me if you didn't. And maybe me getting us started is another ritual.

(F nods, silent)

A: And there's something nice about rituals, as long as they suit how you feel. What would it be like if I didn't start us off?
F: I'd probably say something eventually.
A: Just to break the silence?
F: Yes. Nothing has happened since I was here last, and I don't feel like talking. I'm tired.

(Silence)

A: Tired from?
F: I was up until 11:30 Friday night and got up at 9:00 the next morning, and Saturday I was up until 11:30 again because my parents went to bed, and my sister wanted me to watch Spider Man with her. She said she'd do my chores if I'd watch it with her.

A: That's hysterical, because she wanted your company?

F: Yeah, and there are some parts that are inappropriate, scary for her. And then my mother woke me up at 8:00 am, because we were going somewhere. And I went to bed at 9:30 last night, which is pretty normal, but then having to get up to be at school at 8:00 a.m. and feeling like I have a sleep shortage from the weekend.

A: So, you had a whole backlog of things that you were doing on other people's timing. I know how nice it is for you when it's vacation and you can stay in bed as late as you like.

(Silence)

A: There are things that are important about noticing when you don't feel like talking and when you do. You certainly don't want to feel you have to talk just because.

F: Nods.

A: But at the same time, I think last summer we realised that you were really feeling bad, in part because it was hard to want to talk about all that was troubling you.

F: I think this is different because it's not like I'm feeling really bad.

A: That is different.

(Silence)

F: (I am feeling irritated—like "why do I have to figure out how to get her to communicate?" I don't feel there's something developing in this silence. Rather, that it's a holding pattern, an avoidance pattern, with a bit of, "you can't make me.")

A: I think I could let you be quiet until you felt like talking, but I'm not sure that would be great. One of the things that scared you most was feeling you could not even want to talk to your mother. So, we are trying to find our way... on the one hand you get to not feel like talking, but I think you also don't want me to just leave you with it, without figuring out if the silence is going somewhere.

F: Yes, my mom was getting me up on Sunday to go to shopping. I don't have a bathing suit to go to Barbados.

A: Did you want to do that?

F: Yes, I just didn't want to get up, but we didn't wind up going until later. You never go shopping and buy just one thing. I was in the dressing room with my mom and she kept coming out and saying, 'do you like this hat, do you like these shorts, do you like these sunglasses?' She comes to me for fashion advice. I save her from wearing plaids and stripes or stripes in two different directions.

A: That's funny, you kind of sound like the mom. Or do you ask her for advice too?

F: No, how could she give me advice if I'm the one she gets advice from. The only thing she cares about with my clothes is short shorts. She'll say, 'longer.' Short shorts don't look good on me.

A: Some people like going shopping for bathing suits and some people hate it.

F: I just don't like trying on clothes. I have like three outfits, this one—my uniform - and then jeans and then leggings and then occasionally a dressy dress. I don't really care about fashion, just what I think looks nice. And then my mom buys a thousand things, she's like, 'you need this, sister needs this, dad needs this and then she says, 'we need to make cookies,' so we got cookie mix. She's my aunt. My aunt is always buying things for everyone. My mother didn't used to be like that, but now she is. I watched a film last night. The book was better than the film, but the film was really good too. I'd seen it before, but I noticed something I didn't the first time.

A: What was that?

F: So, the book is narrated by Death. Death knows when everyone will die so it will say things like: 'It's not his time yet.' This town is getting bombed and so everyone is going into some shelter basement. And one family is hiding this Jew in their basement.

A: Where is it set?

F: In Germany, outside of Berlin. And so, when everyone else in the town goes to this shelter the Jew can come out and it's the only time he's been able to see the sky for a long time. That seems like it would be worse than death. The narrator of course isn't really death, it's the author's idea of death. There's one point where the main character's street is bombed, and the name of her street is the German word for heaven. So, they are bombing heaven.

A: And I guess it would be us bombing heaven.

F: Yes, or the British. I wonder whether the author thought of the street as heaven first and then bombing it, or the other way around.

A: It's interesting, lots of time when we're reading, we're in the story, but not so much thinking of the author, but you're wondering how the author imagined the story. We've got to stop.

She puts her drawing in her folder and smiles happily.

Discussion

During the majority of the hour F. does not seem to feel there is any point in talking to me. I think at this point of the treatment she feels safer to be seeing me as she has some sense that I have helped to steer her out of deep waters, but I think it is difficult for her to really feel I could be of any help to her. Despite her seeing little use in talking to me, my comment that she had been left too alone with her emotional life might have reached her and she begins to communicate.

We hear of family experiences when her sister and then her mother want something from her (fashion advice). She expresses comparative indifference to these endeavours and seems to feel some superiority to her mother. Then things deepen with her thoughts about the film. Though it is jarring that she refers to a character as "the Jew", she seems to identify with what it would be like to be shut in and not to see the sky. This reminded me of F.'s fear of being trapped inside the hole, with a shovel instead of a rope.

F.'s preoccupation with death brought to my mind her mother's medical issues before F.'s sister's birth. At one level, F. is struggling with profound issues of death, violence, heaven and hell. At another level, she is rather vacant and feels no one is up to accompanying her. Her parents and I are seen as useless, oblivious objects. A hateful object in some way would be more activating, while F. seems to view her objects as harmless and good, but easy to be superior to. When her objects are useless, she is left alone.

Conclusion

I have found Alvarez's discussion of the stupid object helpful in understanding some children who have little hope of an adult having an interested or interesting mind. I have tried to describe a related concept of children with an oblivious object. It might be difficult for therapists to see how truly oblivious some children might consider adults to be when the child has a conscious attitude of admiration or even idealisation toward his/her parents. When children are in the midst of so much activity and their parents are materially helpful, it can be hard to see how alone they are with their emotional problems. Frances's parents were forced to seek emotional help for their daughter, owing to her level of distress, which they still minimised. Some genuine work took place, and F. was on much more solid ground when she ended treatment a year and a half later. I tried to leave F. with some sense of the importance of her internal life. However, I felt there was a formidable family defense in the direction of activity and success and little sustained parental access to their own internal processes. F. had made real progress, but in some ways, I felt that a status quo had been restored.

As we ended, I let F. know that she had done some hard work to recover her sense of her own individual importance and a deeper understanding of her thoughts and feelings. I am left with the concern that the lessons of this period of F.'s life might feel tempting to forget. A parental need for obliviousness to emotional pain can create children who are oblivious to their own internal worlds. These children's own obliviousness is both an identification with their parents and an avoidance of pain that would be required to see their parents' obliviousness. Such children can look okay until they cannot anymore.

Notes

1   Elsewhere, I have utilised H. Rosenfeld's (1960) conceptualisation of identification with an ill or dead object (Brady, 2016). Green (1983) described a mother still alive, but emotionally unavailable to a child, owing to sudden depression caused by severe loss. The parents I am describing here are alive and well in certain respects, but chronically unavailable to complex or messy emotions in their children.
2   This section is based on Alvarez's (2012) chapter.
3   Bion uses 'mother' to refer to the infant's primary object; it could equally be a father.

References

Alvarez, A. 2012. Issues of narcissism, self-worth and the relation to the stupid object: devalued or unvalued? In: *The Thinking Heart: Three Levels of Psychoanalytic Therapy with Disturbed Children*. Hove and New York: Routledge.

Bion, W.R. 1962. *Learning from Experience*. London: Karnac.

Brady, M.T. 2015. High up on bar stools: manic defences and an oblivious object in a late adolescent. *Journal of Child Psychotherapy*, 41(1): 52–72.

Brady, M.T. 2016. Substance abuse in an adolescent boy: waking the object. *Contemporary Psychoanalysis*, 52(2): 201–223.

Green, A. 1983. The dead mother. In: A. Green. *On Private Madness*. Madison, CT: International Universities Press.

Klein, M. 1946/1975. Notes on some schizoid mechanisms. In: *Envy and Gratitude*. London: The Hogarth Press.

Mondzrak, V. 2012. Reflections on psychoanalytic technique with adolescents today: pseudo-pseudomaturity. *International Journal of Psycho-Analysis*, 93(3): 649–666.

Rosenfeld, H. 1960. On drug addiction. In: *Psychotic States: A Psycho-Analytical Approach*. New York: International Universities Press, pp. 128–143.

Winnicott, D.W. 1958. *The Capacity to be Alone, The Maturational Processes and the Facilitating Environment*. New York: International Universities Press, pp. 29–36.

4 Introjective Processes: Work on the Infantile as a Mental State

Monica Cardenal

Introduction

The geographic perspective of the mind and the emotional dimension of beauty

In the book *Territorios Poskleinianos* (2020) Suzanne Maiello comments that Donald Meltzer was eight years old when his parents took him to Europe for the first time. He was fascinated by the beauty of the construction of its cities and its architecture rich in history. So much so, that he thought of becoming an architect as an adult. Meltzer would say; "To breathe life and beauty into stone seemed to me the highest possible aspiration" (1988, 2020, p. 22) Maiello points out that he became a psychiatrist and psycho-analyst instead, as we all know, but what remained in him was a tendency towards thinking in terms of spaces, interiors and exteriors, as well as of emotional beauty. It might have been that childhood experience of travel-ling with his parents that inspired what would be his developments of the geographic and aesthetic perspective of the mental processes.

The geographic dimension of the mind implies acknowledging that the unconscious mental life takes place in different possible spaces and that, originating in splitting processes of the Self, those spaces will be used for the projection of fantasies in a very concrete way. It was Melanie Klein who, with her psychoanalytic work experience with children towards 1920, started reporting the interest of her young patients in the interior of their own bodies and those of their mothers. Material on prolonged Bick-style infant observations during the first or second years of life shows this infantile interest discovered by Klein in the clinic very vividly. Thus, we owe the notion of projective identification—which was described many years later in 1946—to her. The origin of this idea already appears in the games of Erna (1924), as a type of particular omnipotent fantasy in which a part of the Self can be separated and projected within the object, with enormous consequences for the relationship. Different ways of being inside the object will happen, from the most moderate to the most extreme, in the world of internal relationships, with an effect on the

DOI: 10.4324/9781003246749-4

external ones and the world in general. We acknowledge, therefore, that the idea of spaces and interiorness was revealed by Klein and later developed by Wilfred Bion, Meltzer and Esther Bick, who made novel contributions on human development, psychopathology and clinic starting from this idea sowed by Klein.

Let us start then by considering intrusive and violent projective identification of the Self in the internal object. Meltzer discovered through the clinic a type of process by which the infantile parts of the Self occupy the internal object intrusively, with the aim of trying to resolve anxieties of separation and loss. This intrusive projective identification is the maximum style of defence, which generates confusion between the Self and the object, between internal and external reality, and reverts, for example, the adult-child or analyst—patient bonds, of course with great effects on the transference. In this infantile mental state sadism and destructiveness predominate, the Self sets in motion strategies of deceit, extortion and seduction in its intrusion in the interior of the internal object. In this way, it takes the capacities of the object as its own, not acknowledging that they belong to the object, nor its loving dependence towards it, ultimately, in this infantile sexual state, the Self feels that it owes the internal object nothing. Meltzer will refer to these ideas in his paper on *"The Relation of Anal Masturbation to Projective Identification"* from 1966 and take it up again in *"The psychoanalytic process"* of 1967. It is dedicated to the issue of zonal confusions in the development of the mind, and in consequence, to the psychoanalytic process. In this book he defines five geographic regions: internal—external to the Self, interior and exterior of the object and the no-place of delirious formations. Finally, in *Claustrum,* written in 1992, he consolidates his ideas on the psychopathology of this type of occupation that the Self does in the interior of the internal objects, and in certain compartments. In this book Meltzer talks about six spaces for the mind: the external world, the uterus, the internal world, the interior of the internal objects, the interior of the external objects, and the no-place. Money-Kyrle's contributions (1971) based on these developments are interesting. He links his concept of the spurious substitute of the real object that is no longer remembered to Meltzer's discoveries on anal masturbation and intrusive projective identification. Money-Kyrle explains very well what Meltzer described in 1966, about how babies realise, when discovering and exploring their own rectum, that it evokes the breast at the same time, owing to its shape, and also discover a space which seems to offer an "entrance door" which babies remember they came out of. The result is an extremely confused mental state in which babies are in contact with a substitute for the breast and in projective identification with it within themselves.

Another very particular extreme of defence and splitting is the dismantling of the mind, which leads to de-mentalisation, in which mental activity is temporarily suspended. In the dismantling, which is a desperate strategy to understand the world's functioning, there is no sadism. The Self suffers passively while the attention is disassembled, the senses disperse, no concepts can be generated, and the perception of the passage of time is suspended. In this mental state the emotional experience is not possible, events only occur. For Meltzer, this mental state is linked to the most primitive obsessive mechanisms which operate by separating the sensory experience, and the objects, in order to be able to control them. In the autistic states, the construction of an interior space for the Self, and therefore for the object, does not happen. The object is bi-dimensional. Already in *"Sexual states of the mind"* (1973), Meltzer referred to the dismantling, in which the notion of time and space are noticeably affected. Autistic children have serious difficulties in experimenting and conceptualising a closed, containing space—with sphincters, we might add. Therefore, there is no space in this mental dimension. For the mind the object is so open that it could fall into a vacuum when trying to "get into or enter" it; there is no space to enter. Then the surface-to-surface relationships predominate. This type of identification is adhesive, time is not dimensioned in it. Emotionality is superficial. From that very novel perspective, in order for the projective identification to occur it is necessary to first experiment with an interior space both in the Self and in the object. We owe the discovery of the infantile mental states to Bick and Meltzer, I would add that they are very current discoveries which widen our comprehension of psychopathology in modernity. It is worth mentioning that these ideas led both Bick and Meltzer to change the Kleinian definition of the positions in the development of the human infant. Meltzer understood that the study in the clinic of these primitive states would help understand and reveal the mental processes of early life, probably inaccessible in another kind of patient.

Within this spatial dimension of the mind, we will then add the useful communicative projective identification, as Meltzer considers it, and the introjective identification which enables emotional experience, and leads to the true and intimate bonds. These four types of identifications mentioned here are very well described in the chapter about the Barry case in *"Exploration of autism"* (1975), whose analyst was Doreen Weddell, dedicated to the perturbation of the geography of the vital space in the mind, specifically in cases of autism.

This geographic perspective of the mind is complemented in Meltzer, both in his theory and in his clinic, with the aesthetic perspective, in which the body of the present mother, her face, will set in motion mental processes of vital significance for the development of the personality. This emotional dimension of beauty, which is part of the baby's early world, implies that the apprehension of the mother's beauty and of her interiority, opens the mind to "knowing" and allowing oneself to be impacted by that beauty, without the Self becoming intrusive, quite the opposite. Meltzer talks about an innate response to the beauty of the world (that response contains an integration of Bion's three positive bonds—L, H and K—but the pain in this experience will lead to splitting processes to relieve it) (1986) In this way, infantile sexual states predominate in the mind in which the tolerance to uncertainty and pain, and an ethical positioning will be key in the future of the development of the personality and the bonds. This means that accepting that not everything can be known about the object of love, that there is knowledge that remains veiled to the early Self and is "private" for the object and withstanding not having it entirely is very conflicting and painful. Thus, the early formation of symbols and thoughts become possible, Meltzer even suggests that this happens from the last month of gestation, when the base of these processes is established, and these unfold upon the impact of the mother's body and mind on the external world. This is a possible road to understand the conditions that the mind needs in order to reach those close states known as states of creation, linked to the apprehension of beauty, not as a banal ambition but as a kind of infantile mental state that promotes a subjective transformation, and from there the development of intimate bonds of affection are favoured, the most interesting ones. They are issues that analysts are undoubtedly willing to work on in our consulting rooms.

Meltzer was a specialist in detecting and describing different splitting processes the Self is capable of. Horizontal and vertical divisions, which lead the separated infantile parts - those that have different qualities- to establish ways of relating to the objects from the primary scene in sexual link leading to a range of emotional experiences or to psychopathologies, according to how the internal objects evolve inside the Self on the road to maturity. In "*Sexual states of the mind*" (1973), Meltzer starts reinforcing his theory of compartments of the interior of the maternal body, this maternal interior begins to configure itself according to the personal experience of the child regarding his/her own body orifices and their contents, their fluids, and the exchanges he/she has with the mother, the services she renders: the mouth to the mother's breast, the baby's head to the mother's head and breast, for example. This occurs together with the apprehension of the beauty of the mother and the interest in her interior. At this point, I would like to include the father's mental function dedicated to cleaning the baby's hostilities in the mother's interior, as well as being in charge of feeding her (pregenital oedipal content).

The Introjective Processes: Infant Observation and Psychoanalytic Clinic

Martha Harris wrote: "Introjection remains a mysterious process: how do involved and reliance upon objects in the external world which are apprehended by the senses (and, as Bion has pointed out, described in language which has been evolved to deal with external reality) become assimilated and transformed in the mind into what he calls "psychoanalytic objects" which can contribute to the growth of personality?" (1978, p. 176).

I intend to work on the way in which Infant Observation turns out to be inspiring in order to think about and understand those infantile aspects which we later see vividly present in the transference, both in child analysis and adult analysis. I am interested in highlighting the value of observation for the development of our task as psychoanalysts, where our focus is placed on the transferential processes and their vicissitudes. I wish to link the experience of infant observation to the discoveries in our clinic, a revitalisation of our work as analysts. The observer's role is a place of discovery, something new and unprecedented will happen when a baby is born. We are launched into this experience of allowing ourselves to be impacted by the feelings which are set in motion, so that we can understand them.

Trudy Klauber refers to Bick's method:

"It is an introduction to a new level of understanding, one which is often unspoken, but always present. The baby in the child patient, the child in the adolescent or adult patient- and the significant communication of strong feeling transmitted into the analyst without words".

(2018)

Observation: Roma, two years old, her mother has just had a baby

"...She approached me, she came to sit between us, the mother was breastfeeding the baby. Roma leaned towards me. The baby farted and made a poo, Roma said 'poo' and pointed at her nappy. She lifted her t-shirt and showed her belly. Her mother asked her 'where is your belly?', and she showed her, sucking it in and out, she looked at us, smiling.

...She stood up and took me to the parents' bedroom. I told her it would be dark, but she opened the door and the lamp was on, so I walked behind her and she said 'uck' (for truck) referring to the lamp in that shape. First she went straight to the parents' bed, straightened the sheets as if 'making it', then went to the dresser where the Peppa Pig tin was. She named all the characters, 'S, look!, Peppa, S, look!, George, look! Daddy, cloud, sun'. She took the tin to the bed and back to the dresser, then she went to the crib, took a baby perfume that was there and said 'perfume'. She put it down and went to the parents' bathroom, I followed her, she took up a bar of soap 'oap', she said and put it back. Later she began to jump with both feet together and said: 'Jump, S!', and I had to do the same".[1]

Roma never appears to be hostile or intrusive, quite the opposite, her curiosity is creative and full of significance; she manifests a careful interest in her parents' bedroom, their bed and personal, intimate objects. She wants to enter that world of relationships which express intimacy. The room is dark, but she dares to enter that interior. As regards her parents' objects, I believe she appreciates their beauty, their smell, she picks soaps and perfumes. It means that she is interested in the interior of the parental couple in relation and in the baby, their principal and most exciting creation. From there she talks, she communicates with the observer about this. She evokes her "papa". She is so interested in what occurs between them that she is capable of "smoothing their sheets", in that way being the dedicated and considerate daughter. Perhaps there is a minimal manic atmosphere towards the end of the sequence, let us take into account that she is a small child, and she is emotionally going through many significant experiences, she does not avoid pain. She preferred to show the observer all her interest in each of the objects belonging to her parents, including the baby—undoubtedly the most precious object—but without stealing them, without becoming intrusive. Maybe the presence of the observer helps her to digest the feelings of pain and exclusion because of her brother's birth. In this way, Roma, just as she fantasise about the baby, feels received in the mind of a loving object like the observer, who has known her since she was born. Let us take into account, too, that this happen after withstanding having to see her mother breastfeed the baby. How many fantasies referring to body contents, and the interior of her body, the baby's and her mother's were set in motion? Perhaps the "belly dance" is the clearest evidence of this spatial dimension as a way of understanding the world of internal and external relationships, separation processes, feelings of exclusion, the arrival of another baby, the parents' sexuality…

Tolerating the inevitable pain that results from exclusion, especially in reference to the relationship between the parents, and its creative products - babies- allows the Self to achieve the necessary mental state to develop thoughts and emotions and be grateful for that possibility. It knows, acknowledges, that this capacity is due to its own internal objects; acknowledges and that its internal creative capacities and thoughts have been inspired by its internal objects. This is the process of introjective identification described by Meltzer. As we can see, the mind is in condition to reach those infantile sexual states very early in the development (Cardenal, 2014).

Literature, dreams, oniric thoughts

17-year-old Francesco arrived at the consultation totally depressed. His parents were foreigners and the family included three more sons. It was not only impossible for him to think, he also had enormous difficulties when being in contact with others, closeness even generated an unbearable claustrophobic experience in him. His daily life was plagued with obsessive controls. He could not use public transport or circulate wherever there were other people who could brush past him. Certain noises were unbearable to him, noises which would be imperceptible to other people. That anguish was experienced at physical level, his body tensed, his muscles hardened, and he remained paralysed without saying a word in front of others. Claustrophobic episodes, with sensory predominance, occurred daily, the symbolic mental plane was clearly affected. Emotional life seemed still, I always got the impression that they were not attacks to the bond in the Bionian style, but a clear difficulty in understanding the world symbolically, of course his capacity for insight was also very poor in the early stages of treatment. The infantile Self- cloistered perhaps inside an internal mother- inhabiting his head and chest seemed to feel sheltered in this way from any rivalry and oedipal danger, with the fantasy of keeping the destructive and dissociated infantile aspects at bay. Perhaps Francesco had a constant fear of being caught out as an intruder. The interest, fundamentally of his infantile part, seemed to be the ability to remain inside a part of his internal mother, sheltered. We could add, therefore, that this confinement might also offer him the defensive fantasy of keeping the sadistic Superego under control. Francesco had been an over-adapted child, too proper, and an excellent student until he became depressed, I would insist, in an infantile way.

Francesco read fiction, at the beginning tales of death and desolation. Those stories had a poor literary construction. The themes referred especially to reformatories and juvenile boarding schools (the Claustrum) and were seldom brought to the session; I would say that they were read in "private" behind closed doors. Francesco practically did not speak.

After a time in analysis, where the central focus was on paternal transference, to my surprise he started to become inclined towards creative literature of higher quality, among the books he chose was *The New York Trilogy* by Paul Auster, in which one of the stories is about a father locking his son up and removing him from any possibility of "language", so that he can speak his "true language", while a depressed poet "detective", burdened by his grief and madness, tries to investigate the case. Aspects of himself came into play; his interest—and later my interest—in Literature gave us the possibility to analyse them. Francesco himself led the way and I followed, as an analyst, and always "read" the book that the patient narrated, none other.

Little by little Francesco no longer read "silently", he brought the books and the thoughts and emotions they evoked in him as material for analysis. My interest was surely perceived by him, he was no longer depressed and avoidant, but was willing to "go into" his interest towards me. At the same time there started to appear with increasing frequency brief dreams about jungle animals with a clear oedipal content, they were very entertaining dreams for me, and transparent like those of young children. Dreams about snakes, crocodiles, big cats, the setting was almost always the jungle. The internal landscape had changed from the desolate desertic silence to the "exuberant vegetation" he used to describe in his dreams. His infantile parts were less scared of updating some of the early contact with his mother as an object of beauty, a landscape which one yearns to know, not without conflict. At this stage of the treatment Francesco not only talked more and dreamed, but also was much less avoidant with the world of relationships and his obsessions had noticeably subsided.

An aesthetic perspective was opening new roads for the mind, and I believe this was possible, owing to the analytical device. A geographic distribution of fantasies was perhaps beginning to define an interior and exterior of the body and mind in a clearer way, in the Self and in the object. And the words could then circulate with more "rhythm". When he was able to speak fluently in the session, he told me that he realised now that he had not spoken before because he felt very confused in his thoughts and was afraid of confusing the others.

As he began to speak more, although he brought few dreams and lots of books to the session, a dream he brought repeatedly was one in which he was in a library. He generally described different types of rooms and doors that he would pass by and open into that space full of books in which he was interested and fascinated by. Sometimes the books were on a "top floor" and the rooms would have ladders and different colours on the walls. The doors would open, leading from one book-filled room to another. To me, it was a very significant and aesthetic kind of dream. Once again spaces and inner landscapes, a fascination of books and their mysterious contents to be discovered. The creative imagination was emerging, so linked to the interior of a mother whose "meaning" (knowledge) started to interest him and he no longer thought of avoiding. An interior filled with books and colours is not just any interior, I insist that something was being revitalised.

The Writer and his Ghosts (1963), by the renowned Argentinian writer Ernesto Sabato, is a book which the author dedicated to his mother and which Francesco brought to analysis, with much interest. The patient commented that in that book Sabato was seeking human subjectivity through literature and language, telling me that the fact that we spoke about the same things in the sessions had caught his attention, and that "we used" many of the words Sabato used. I was not the only one who used those words, there was a plural. Possibly, he was the writer with a background in physics and mathematics just like Sabato, and who was now greatly interested in the words and their manifestation in the links.

The beauty of words and their bonding possibility were being discovered by Francesco's inner child. His unconscious baby parts were interested in my interest in his books. The little poet detective Auster was in the midst of subjective work and I, his analyst, enjoyed his capacity for creative investigation displayed in transference. The landscapes had changed in my patient's inner world, and, to him, in my interior.

Note

1   I am grateful to Silvia De Egea for the observation material which I supervised for two years.

References

Bick, E. 1963. Notas sobre la observación de lactantes en la enseñanza del psicoanálisis. *Revista de Psicoanálisis*, Vol. XXIV.

Bick, E. 1968. The Experience of the Skin in Early Object Relations. In: Harris Williams, M., ed. *Collected Papers of Martha Harris and Esther Bick*. The Roland Harris Trust.

Bion, W.R. 1962. *Learning from Experience*. London: Karnac.

Bion, W.R. 1967. *Volviendo a pensar*. Buenos Aires: Editorial Lumen-Hormé.

Cardenal, M. 2014. Belleza, creación, misterio. El conflicto estético. *Revista de Psicoanálisis de Guadalajara*, vol. 9, 2015.

Ferrater Mora, J. 1958. *Diccionario de Filosofía*. Buenos Aires: Editorial Sudamericana.

Harris, M. 1978. Towards learning from experience in infancy and childhood. In: *Collected paper of Martha Harris and Esther Bick*, ed. Meg Harris Williams, Karnac.

Klauber, T. (2018) Editorial. *Revista Internacional de Observación de bebés*, Vol. 1, ed. Monica Cardenal and Jeanne Magagna, Gradiva.

Klein, M. 1932. Neurosis obsesiva en una niña de 6 años, en *El Psicoanálisis de niños*, ed. Paidós, Buenos Aires.

Klein, M. 1946. Notes on some schizoid Mechanisms. In: *The Writings of Melanie Klein*.

Maiello, S. 2020. Explorando las dimensiones espaciales de la mente. In: *Territorios poskelinianos. Una actualización de la tarea psicoanalítica*. ed. Cardenal, M. and Redonda, M. Buenos Aires: Editorial Teseo.

Meltzer, D. 1966. The Relation of Anal Masturbation to Projective Identification. *International Journal of Psycho-Analysis.*, 47(2–3), pp. 335–342.

Meltzer, D. 1967. *The Psychoanalytical Process*. London: Heinemann.

Meltzer, D. 1975. *Explorations in Autism*. London: Clunie Press.

Meltzer, D. et al. 1986. *Studies in extended Metapsychology –Clinical Applications of Bion's Ideas*. The Roland Harris Educational Trust.

Meltzer, D. and Harris Williams, M. 1988. *The Apprehension of Beauty –The Role of aesthetic Conflict in Development, Art and Violence*. The Roland Harris Trust Library.

Meltzer, D. 1992. *Claustrum. Una investigación de los fenómenos claustrofóbicos*. Buenos Aires: Spatia.

Money-Kyrle, R. 1971. The Aim of Psycho- Analysis. In: *The collected papers of Roger Money-Kyrle*. Edited by Meltzer, D. with the assistance of O'Shaughnessy, E. Clunie Press.

5 The Interpretation of Oedipal Configurations in Child Analysis

Florence Guignard

When a child analyst says that he is listening to an "oedipal material", what does he mean?

By discovering the stages of the psychosexual development—oral, anal, phallic and genital—Freud (1905) established a first series of parameters he never later disavowed. Let us also remember the developments brought to this series by Karl Abraham (1924).

On the other hand, the concept of the "Oedipus Complex", which was implicit since Freud's first letters to Fliess (1887–1902) took its almost definitive shape in 1910. Organised around the fourth year of life, the Oedipus Complex will find its "resolution" (1924) in a set of identifications to the objects of oedipal desires that the child has to give up as such, equally on the direct as on the inverted side of this Complex.

However, between those two series of parameters—stages of libidinal development on the one hand, and differentiation between "pre-oedipal" and "oedipal" on the other—the links are not always easy to establish: there is, in particular, often a confusion between "pre-oedipal" and "pre-genital".

In addition to this, let us remember that Freud considered "infantile genital sexuality" (1923) as being organised under the primacy of "phallicity"—and therefore, as unisex. This consideration is contrary to his description of the criteria of the resolution of the Oedipus Complex, in which he includes an acknowledgement both of the difference of sexes and of generations.

We meet here two central problems, not only from a theoretical point of view, but also from that of understanding the clinical material, and choosing the right technical means, particularly in the field of *interpretation*:

The first problem is that of the *nature of the drives*, as, according to Freud, *libido is of male essence*.

The second problem is the fact that the *biological bedrock* lies, according to Freud, in the *repudiation of femininity in both sexes* (1937).

Last, not least, the Freudian developments on *primal fantasy* (1914–18 and 1915) confront us with another parameter, as, through its four aspects, Freud establishes the primacy of a genital fantasy from the very beginning of psychic life, if not from a phylogenetic inheritance.

DOI: 10.4324/9781003246749-5

I proposed (1996–2020) to consider that the four aspects of primal fantasy are paired two by two in a relation of *reciprocal inclusion: the fantasy of coming back to intra-uterine life* pairing with *the fantasy of castration* on the one hand, and *the fantasy of seduction* pairing with the *fantasy of primal scene* on the other hand. In clinical material, these fantasmatic aspects would play their parts as *defensive formations against the four components of human destiny: birth, biological sex determination, constant pressure of drives and difference of generations.*

Thus, *fantasy of coming back to intra-uterine life* would be used as a *denial of being born; fantasy of castration* would constitute its complementary version, as a *denial of biological sex determination. Fantasy of seduction* would play its part as a *denial of the constant pressure of drives,* in a relation of reciprocal inclusion with the *fantasy of the primal scene,* which expresses the *denial of the difference of generations.*

Counter to both the persisting dichotomy between *pre-oedipal* and *oedipal,* and the Freudian primacy of phallicity, Melanie Klein's clinical work brought her to observe and conceptualise an early version of the oedipal configuration (1928). This early version occurs, for the baby, in the immediate footstep of its discovery of otherness, discovery that Klein would later develop under the term of *depressive position* (1931).

Linked to her masterly description of the psycho-sexual development of girl and boy (1932), this early version of an oedipal configuration inevitably brings every psychoanalyst—be he child analyst or adult analyst—to reconsider a series of technical and theoretical parameters in his daily clinical work. In fact, taking into account that genital drives become active during the period of "exacerbation of sadism"—a period that will later be considered as *the threshold of the depressive position*—Melanie Klein establishes what she calls *the early feminine phase.* It is worth remembering that she considers this phase as occurring in both girls *and* boys, and that she describes it as consisting of an identification—*projective identification,* we might say nowadays—of the baby to the desire of the mother for the father and his penis. She values this early feminine phase as being a privileged internal space for developing the capacity for introjection; from the point of view of psychopathology, she considers it as being the fixation point of male homosexuality.

I named (1987) *"primal maternal space"* the earliest configuration of a relationship in which the new-born establishes its projective identification to the "capacity of reverie" (Bion) of the mother, (1961), and *"primal feminine space"* the part of psychic space where the "early feminine phase" appears later on. In linking these two primal organisations of psychic space, we obtain the parameters that will allow the early oedipal configuration to occur in its twofold aspect: direct and inverted.

When the analyst works with young children, the representation he can have of these different parameters will obviously be of utmost importance, as he will be confronted with the choice of both the *level* and the *format* of his interpretations.

I propose to develop here the questions raised by the work of the psychoanalyst with very young children, through a short, classical, almost emblematic clinical vignette:

Paul, nearly three years old, rushes into the consulting room, gets hold of the doll's dinner and of the modelling clay, and invites his (female) analyst to a private dinner; he refuses with great energy the idea of other "toy-people" coming and sharing this "meal". He pours water into two cups, generously watering the whole table in the same movement, makes sausages and pancakes with the clay, gives his therapist some to "eat", "eats" some himself? He then vigorously plants a small stick into one of the pancakes. But the stick breaks inadvertently… Paul stops at once, examines the break, looks at the therapist with a puzzled face. She looks back at him with a silent, attentive face. Paul chooses the biggest part of the broken stick and goes on pushing it into the clay; he does so with as much determination as before, but with more concentration and application. He now observes, like an artist, the hollows made in the clay and, with supreme attention, delicately takes a small pebble that happens to be lying around and puts it into one of the hollows. As the analyst is still held by the delight of what she understands, logically enough, as the expression of Paul's desire to make a baby with her, the little boy gets hold of the clay pancake, throws it on the floor, stamps on it, then sits on it and squashes it thoroughly with his bottom, wriggling and uttering suggestive noises of defecation. Then, with a languishing demeanour, he goes to the toy box, chooses a little rag-doll, and lies down on the couch with the doll on his heart, sucking his thumb.

This scene occurs in the first session after a weekend; Paul has had about three months of therapy, three times a week. It has probably been understood that Paul is not a psychotic child. I shall deliberately refrain from saying anything more about his pathology or his history.

How can we understand, along classical Freudian lines, this rather ordinary way of playing? Is it an oedipal desire to have sex, to fertilise, and to give birth? And if so, is it with the mother, or with the father? Or is it a pre-oedipal desire? And if so, how can one characterise Paul's more or less sadistic oral, anal, urethral and phallic drives? What is the nature of his desire: desire to incorporate the breast and the penis? expression of love for the maternal mother? for the sexual mother? for the fertilising father? What is his desire linked to? To troubles in feeding (and here we would have to introduce data foreign to the transference-countertransference situation)? Or to topographical regression, linked, according to Freud, to the adult analytical setting of the couch (and here we would be confronted with the discussion of similarities and differences between adult and child analytic treatment)? What is the economic function of Paul's primal fantasies in the *hic et nunc* of that session, after the weekend separation? How do we grasp the dynamics that runs among the different aspects of human destiny, actualised in the transference relationship and denied through the fantasmatic expression of playing?

Indeed, the Kleinian point of view on early oedipal configurations is of considerable help to understand this "private dinner" and to resolve, by overcoming it, the alternatives I have just put forward, i.e.: pre-oedipal or oedipal? We can understand that, playing this "private dinner" allows Paul not only to develop, in the analytic space, the problematics of loss of the primary object and his efforts towards anal and phallic control, but also to express *simultaneously* a sexual and directly genital desire for his analyst, with the castration problematics associated to it. The anal and urethral components of his oedipal configuration appear, both in his making suggestive sausages, and in his generously spreading water; his desire for phallic domination is expressed through his introducing the stick into the play; his castration anxieties are present when he breaks that stick. All the levels of infantile sexuality are thus expressed in this picture of "little Oedipus before the classical Freudian Oedipus".

However, this will not rid us of our difficulties:

- On the one hand, the last part of the game has not yet been examined in my previous remarks: what can we think of this defecating/giving birth to a "baby" that seems to quieten and satisfy this little boy's drives?
- On the other hand, the relatively easy understanding of this material doesn't give us the slightest guarantee of the quality of the *interpretation* of it. Certainly, this interpretation will be worth being spoken of only if it is given *in the transference*, and you might object that this condition should supply the answer to my theoretical questions and appease my worries. It is not my opinion, for the simple reason that nothing is more difficult than to express feelings and desires—see art and literature—and that both a particular gift and a good training are required, in order to put into words desires and feelings which are addressed to the analyst, as a representative of somebody else, the patient himself being unaware of this displacement.

Edmond Rostand's *Cyrano de Bergerac* offers a fairly good metaphor for the transference situation: *Christian*, a pleasant but very inhibited young man who is *Roxane*'s object of love, might represent her idealised paternal object; moreover, he will soon disappear from the scene, being killed in battle. *Cyrano*, an oldish man, ugly and witty, might well represent the psychoanalyst at work: he will respect Roxane until death, in spite of his loving feelings for her; and, putting his spirit in the service of the passion she feels for Christian, he will lend his voice to this latter, who will thus be able to conquer Roxane during "the balcony scene". In the same way our patients depart when their analysis is over, given back to their oedipal destiny which has been clarified by means of the analytic work. This metaphor is even more appropriate in child analysis, as children are still living with the vital necessity of keeping good enough relationships with their family environment, in order to be able to survive and develop, in conditions totally out of their control.

In order to go further on the way of *interpretation*, let us now complicate the problem a little more:

- First of all, let us replace *Paul* by a hypothetical *Paula*, still in the same scene, and still with a woman analyst. What about *Paula*'s genital desires? Will she project her father onto the analyst, regardless of the analyst's sex, or shall we have to think of predominantly homosexual desires, on the inverted side of her oedipal configuration? Or else, do we have to understand, in her playing of the "private dinner", a purely oral expression of her desires for the breast, considering those as *pre-oedipal* desires? Wouldn't we thus be complying with our unconscious refusal of the genital infantile sexuality? And how should we understand her play with the clay? Will the anal component be alone on the stage? If not, which of the three components of the equation *penis-baby-faeces* will have a predominant meaning at that precise moment in the treatment? Will the spreading of water and the use of the stick have to be understood as a phallic claim? And if so, shall we deduce from it that *Paula* is exemplifying by this means a *unisex, phallic infantile sexual theory*? Fortunately, and contrary to the situation with *Paul*, the end of the sequence could be seen as totally congruent with the feminine way of functioning...

Before coming back to these questions from the point of view of identifications, I would like to push the speculation as far as possible, imagining now that the same scene happens with a male analyst, first for *Paul*, then for *Paula*... How should we reorganise the understanding of all the parameters described above? Should we suppose that *Paul*'s homosexual tendencies prevailed in a pathological way, while *Paula* appeared as the pure model of normality? *Last, not least*, what use could have this game in the psychoanalytic process?

To these many queries, the problematics of *identification* will bring many answers which, in turn, will reveal even more complex aspects of the question.

We know that Freud pointed to identification as being the first mode of object relations (1921). However, he left uncertain both the characteristics of this early identification/relation, and the links of analogy—or opposition—that this latter could have with the secondary, post-oedipal identifications. Melanie Klein fills the gap by proposing much more precise parameters, with the concept of *part object* (1931) on the one hand, and with the development of the concept of *projective identification* on the other hand (1946) brilliantly completed and extended by Bion (1961).

Nevertheless, in the spiral of the discoveries about human psyche, amplitude and complexity of identificatory organisation brings with it the possibility of using this very organisation for defensive purposes.

Let us take an example: how can we articulate the oedipal desires, both genital *and* pre-genital, of *Paul* and/or *Paula*, with his/her projective identification to the female analyst or male analyst? Should we understand the playing at dinners as a metaphorical expression of the situation of "psychic feeding" offered by the analyst—and thus place this latter as a maternal-mothering object in the transference, regardless to his/her sexual identity? Or should we also take into account the genital aspects of the oedipal dimension, with primal scene fantasy exacerbated by the weekend separation? And, in this case, what shape should the interpretation of that primal scene take? Should one suggest to the child that he/she brings to the stage what he/she imagines has happened to the analyst with a "third person", during the separation? And if so, which kind of scene, and with which "third person"? Daddy feeding Mummy with good things? But in that case, the early genital drives would be evacuated from the interpretation, to the great relief of the analyst's Superego, but at the expense of the accurateness of understanding of the child's drive movements?

I already hear the objections to my way of putting things, especially the idea that, at least with a non-psychotic child, one cannot expect the same material to come up, whether boy or girl, and whether the analyst be a man or a woman.

This is precisely one of the parameters I want to display in my reflection on the interpretation of oedipal configurations, both with adults and children patients. My opinion is that any material obtained in a session, whether oedipal or not, will not only vary according to the patient's pathology; it will also depend on the following variables:

- patient's gender;
- analyst's gender;
- quality of the patient's basic psychic identity, whether a boy or a girl, a man or a woman;
- quality of the analyst's basic psychic identity, whether a man or a woman;
- prevalence, in the patient, of projective processes over introjective ones, or vice versa;
- prevalence, in the analyst, of projective processes over introjective ones, or vice and versa;
- normality or pathology of projective identification in the patient;
- normality or pathology of projective identification in the analyst.

To conclude, I would propose the idea that, even with a very young child, it is the meeting of the analyst's *Infantile* [1] and the analysand's *Infantile* that builds up the *internal framework* of the analytic situation. Simultaneously, this meeting accounts for the *blind spots* that occur in one, or the other, or both protagonists of the analytic treatment.

As analysts, we have the responsibility of the functioning of our psychic apparatus during the session, including the unconscious aspects of it. Hence, we have to pay a particularly careful attention to our *blind spots*, of which we have only indirect information, as they are, by definition, unconscious.

It is probably *the urge to interpret* that should first warn us, particularly when the interpretation coming into our mind seems brightly obvious to us. In my opinion, it is absolutely necessary to *disjoin* the urge we feel to intervene, from the content of the interpretation that seems so evident to us. I have often asserted that an "obvious interpretation" frequently constitutes what I call a *plug-interpretation*, which is one of the most reliable indications that something defensive is happening in our countertransference, a *blind spot* at the level of our own *Infantile*.

Self-analysis *in situ* is the only means we have at hand to try and evaluate the *nature* of this urge to speak: is it an urge coming from our own *Infantile* and only from it? Or is it an *insight* into the helplessness of the patient's *Infantile*? In this latter case, we could well find ourselves at one of those privileged meeting points between the two *Infantile*—ours and that of the patient. From such meeting points, it is indeed necessary to intervene, not with an interpretation of content nor with a direct transfer interpretation, but by means of a delicate search to put into words the *emotion* in question.

According to my experience, this situation happens even more frequently in analysis with children and adolescents than with adults. Here is the supreme point of the difficulty and the pleasure of our profession as psychoanalysts.

Note

1 For the exact meaning of that concept, see Guignard, F.: The Infantile in the analytic relationship, *International Journal of Psychoanalysis.*, vol. 76, part 4, 1996 and *The Infantile in Psychoanalytic Practice Today*, published in 2022 by Karnac.

6 Secrecy in the Infantile...

Julieta Alejandra Paglini

Contextualising in contemporary times

Contemporary society is undergoing historical, cultural and social changes. Technology has made incoercible advances that increase differences while conveying complexities beyond the understanding of a large majority of the population. Violence is currently one of the principal modes of affective expression, resulting from a low tolerance towards frustration, dissent, differences with others…

The fall of ideals leads to questioning and disregarding some rules of culture, and this has an effect not only on subjectivity, but also on the ways of structuring the psychism. Difficulties are recorded in the establishment of the parameters of temporality, which often appear in the clinic as the experience of an eternal present. These changes inevitably have consequences for our clinical practice.

There is no subjectivity that can be isolated from culture and social life, nor is there a culture that can be detached from the subjectivity that sustains it.

We are immersed in a society that idolises consumption and immediacy, as ways of offering shortcuts to silence emotions; this sometimes involves impoverishing human bonds.

Seemingly easy, surely quick paths, with the "illusion" of being able to deny the signs of the emotional, in an attempt to cover up shortcomings inherent to the human.

The aim is the avoidance of pain, in a quest to fill those gaps with epochal market offers, creating a utopia of completeness.

Zygmunt Bauman describes today's society as a liquid modernity. The liquid is formless. It takes the form of its container. If there is no container, the liquid is drained.

Time is lived in a vertiginous manner; an a-historical way of acting is promoted with a view to invalidating the flow of time. To annul the uncertainty that characterises life, to cover anguish?

Eternal present, eternal youth? The denial of the finiteness of the human being.

DOI: 10.4324/9781003246749-6

The predominance of doing, over thinking and feeling, as a way of dealing with frustration.

Establishing an illusory space of pleasure, of narcissistic brightness, of comfort, where, apparently, conflict disappears.

In the age of communication, of social networks, of a hyper-connected world, what place does intimacy occupy? Could this mode of exchange hinder the recognition of others?

Everyday problems inherent to life itself are pathologised. Anguishes and discontents that in the past were just moments to be experienced, are now being treated with medications. It seems that the phenomenon of the medicalisation of life goes hand in hand with contemporary subjectivity.

In this context, we find parents who confuse love with freedom, who do not set boundaries, without realising that limits according to the age and needs of the children are fundamental in order to build themselves as subjects. If children lack boundaries, how can they incorporate norms? We are witnessing the suppression of generational differences.

Suddenly the impact of the unexpected, the pandemic, COVID-19 spread all over the world. A situation that imposes on us the need to question psychoanalysis, the clinic, and theory. We had to establish new ways of daily practice, and we started to use other tools.

2020 and the pandemic have led us to revisit *Civilization and Its Discontents*, written almost 100 years ago by Freud. Today, the epidemiological situation requires us to distance ourselves from others.

Freud told us that the more culture grows, the greater the uneasiness. The discomfort caused by COVID-19, hand in hand with unpredictability, comes at a time when the human being rejects discomfort and quick satisfaction becomes the order of the day.

Discomfort and its various forms: fear, uncertainty, anguish, experience of emptiness, bodily illnesses, depression, terrors, among others. COVID-19 confronts us with helplessness, with the most human thing we have as humans; the helplessness with which we come into the world.

What a short time ago was thought of as an occasional praxis has now been imposed as the only possible way of sustaining the encounter with the patients.

We wonder what of the specificity of our psychoanalytic practice is sustained and what is "lost". Is it lost? What of the subjectivities is modified in this instance of "confinement"? What does this new situation, that affects through globalisation, the whole world, unleash in each person? Do they change? Perhaps we should wait for this situation to pass, in order to come closer to an answer in the future.

Patients and analysts find themselves facing the same reality.

The challenge lies in taking the necessary time to allow thought and word to predominate over action, the rescue of singularity, of the case by case over the homogenisation of consumption, tolerating the uncertainty of the ups and downs of the clinical work, recognising the traces that the epochal moment leaves behind. Those that promote changes in the subjectivity of each individual.

How are we working today? Clinical work requires trying to set up a particular device for each patient wishing to install an analytical process.

The secret in the infantile...

Why did I choose this title? My desire to write about secrecy was inspired by my practice with children on the margins of puberty-adolescence who experienced suffering as intolerable.

Secret, according to the Real Academia Española (Royal Spanish Academy) comes from the Latin *secrētum*, which is "something that is carefully kept secret and hidden" and also a "mystery (something that cannot be understood)".

Let us think of the birth of a child, a being different from the parents. It seems obvious, but the birth of a child implies the recognition of a subject other than the mother and the father. It is the birth of another life, the enigma of human life. Would it be some sort of secret, a mystery that cannot be unveiled?

The human being is the only creature that comes into the world totally helpless. Its original defencelessness imposes that loving parents welcome the child and take care of its body in the very first encounters while making it possible for it to transmute into an erogenous body. The founding moment that will enable inscriptions, transcriptions, re-transcriptions, elaborations, creations... Thanks to the libidinal bath of language and love the baby becomes a subject susceptible to emotionality, desires, budding thoughts.

Defencelessness, a mark through which the subject, in order to access desire, needs to be desired and loved, and at the same time supported by the other. Fundamental encounter with the lap and the libidinising voice of the others in order to be able to inscribe and link one's own traces.

We think of helplessness as a structuring feature, without it the *infans* would not become a subject. Defencelessness that drives and pushes towards the construction of the subject. What is particularly human is the prolonged need for the assistance of others, at the same time this other satisfies these needs, desires, this other who is endowed with an unconscious, with a veiled place of mind. The subject does not know about itself, a secret?

The baby is thrown into the adventure of the presence and absence of the object. Thanks to them, the first psychic act takes place; hallucination inaugurates the psyche through the experience of satisfaction. Mythical moment, founding of the psychic apparatus. The infant, in his impulse to make up for what he lacks, precariously encounters the limit.

The very first inscriptions that will make their mark, and the absence of the object, an emptiness that pushes it to transcribe and re-transcribe what it has experienced and perceived, inaugurating the thing-presentation overdetermined by cenesthesis, olfactory, visual, sensory perceptions... Marks in a process of tense activity, of intense psychic work.

A structuring traumatic situation, primary violence, in Piera Aulagnier's words. The object is absent, it imposes excesses necessary for the foetus to become human, adult-child asymmetry, the need of the other for living, for being. The object is there, and then, it is not there, at the same time as it overexcites, (without knowing it), it imposes excesses, traumatic excesses as a mark on the selvedge of each individual.

Each subject will deal with traumatism in two stages and in a unique and unrepeatable way. Traumatism is re-signified, re-transcribed via *Nachträglich*. It is the writing of the subject's history in an open temporality in order to flow forward and backward. In this way it gives another meaning to what has been experienced from a different perspective, in the light of the present moment.

We emphasise the importance of the object in this laborious path of the constitution of the subject. In order to access desire, it is indispensable for the baby to have been desired, highlighting as indispensable a certain degree of frustration in this encounter with the other, who limits, who acts as a frontier, a motor for the inauguration of hallucination as the first psychic act.

We have, so far, made an attempt to explain the reasons behind secrecy in the infantile. On the one hand, the defencelessness of the biological body and, on the other hand, the necessary dependence of the infant on the other's culture, on the other, who libidinises.

In order for a child to become a child, is it not necessary for the infant to be able to keep representations, thoughts, fantasies hidden, reserved, shrouded, in mystery? Thinking contains the seed of being able to choose between the thoughts that the person wishes to transmit and which of them to keep secret.

We understand that a certain opacity of the mind is fundamental for the construction of subjectivity; the unconscious is the most intimate secret of the subject.

The secret sets a limit, promotes thought, fantasy, symbolisation. The child needs autonomy, to be distinguished from the "other". The "no" implies the I-other differentiation. Separation of subject from object and vice versa.

To think in secret, in silence, in solitude, with pleasure, without having to share one's thoughts, is obviously a psychic act in its own right.

The clinic

Patients consult us because they are suffering. Their hurt tells us that their defences, their possibilities of re-signifying, their anguishes and conflicts have failed.

We depart from the assumption that in the analytic space we "listen" to our patients without theoretical pre-conceptualisations, a space to be built between the two members of the analytic couple, with the particularity that, when we work with children, adolescents or teenagers, parents also participate directly or indirectly.

In this field participants can be generous or narcissistic parents, children with concerns, anxieties, fears, voids, turbulences, sufferings, anguishes, etc., and the analyst. All these elements will build a net where drives, words, emotions, acts and games will unfold in an associative dynamic, stirring up emotions and phantasmatic, which intervene like a compass in our work, giving us insight into the psychic functioning of the child and its representations, creations, thoughts, feelings, expressions, voids, pains, secrets, silences...

Pubescent children find themselves on the road to exogamy, not at all easy, leaving the small world of the family group to meet their peers. New spaces, new models, a founding moment of turbulent movements, a new meaning to what has been lived, what has been represented. New thoughts, positions, cathexes and decathexes are born. Symbolic wefts are woven and at the same time unwoven, it is a time of intense psychic work. The loss of known places, the entrance to unknown ones; the crossing towards symbolisations and representations. Unconscious mesh where new ways are interwoven.

Vignette

The suffering of the person I will call X became so unbearable that it led him to reveal part of a secret to his mother who, together with his father, offered him to consult a psychoanalyst... X took it decisively and without hesitation.

X told his mother in tears: "I have a horrible thought, which is about death. I want to go back to your belly, to being a child".

X's parents were concerned, so they consulted. X was in the transition from puberty to adolescence.

X said: "I don't get as excited as I used to, my emotions don't vibrate as much as my body. There are times when my mind is blank, literally blank, just thinking about what I see, as if I couldn't remember my thoughts. I feel as if my mind did not work properly. I can't remember what I was doing before because it doesn't matter, it's gone. That brings me a lot of uneasiness and a lot of pressure, I can't concentrate, I don't have a goal, a dream".

X perceived bodily and emotional changes in him, feelings of strangeness, emptiness, loss. He finished primary school, changed classmates and spaces, and at the same time his body and mind changed. He was scared, he did not recognise himself. Oblivion came, by means of repression? invasion of quantity that sweeps away? Thrown into open spaces he experienced the search for himself as a subject, for his sexed way of being, which makes the transition from infancy to adolescence a fearful one.

X: "When I say something I think that it is not really what I want to say, it is very heavy to want to say something and not be able to say it. Anguish keeps me closed and doesn't let me do anything, it is a strange thought, it's not comfortable, I don't feel safe, it's very heavy. Nothing cheers me up, really, I don't feel adrenaline in my body like I did a year ago, I don't have the same energy, the only thing I do is lay in bed. I don't like being with a lot of people like I used to, I don't enjoy socialising as much. It's very difficult for me to detach myself from who I was before, I feel that adolescence is going to be very difficult, it's not fun, it's going to be an unhappy growth. It's very difficult for me to encourage myself to look for other things. I feel very insecure, as if everything is a dream or a hallucination, or nothing is real because everything is sad and distressing".

Transference with the analyst provides the space for the construction of a desiderative net.

X: "I feel very good when I talk".

And he revealed his secret: "The internet is full of bad things. When I was 12 years old I saw a video in which a girl killed herself and the music at the end brought me a lot of anguish. Every time that music plays it makes me sad. It's like horror music. The most terrifying thing was that the girl was my age. It made me very insecure. My sensitivity was hurt, something happened to me since then. The strange thing is that I saw the video in September 2018 and it affected me in a delayed way, in October 2019".

He saw the video of the suicide, the death of a teenager, and kept that image, that music, that terror. He kept his secret hidden, in the darkness until he gave way to a new moment in his life. Loss, pain, strangeness, it was in the analysis where X was able to unfold the uncanny phantasmatic of the transit, of the transformation from worm to butterfly, from child to adolescent.

The present drives to the work of elaboration, re-elaboration, resignification of traces a posteriori and representations, allowing to imagine a project, a future to be constructed as a desiring potentiality.

In the consulting room, in transference with his analyst, X could express something that he saw as another place, the place of being a man and entering the world of men.

It was the body of X that drew him near to some enigmas about growth.

In the accompaniment with his analyst, he invented, or reinvented? the possibility of elaborating the anguish of the present in another way. As if the invisible light of the present cast its shadow on the past, and the past, touched by that shadow thread, acquired the capacity to respond to the darkness of the present.

X: "I feel better, I've spent a lot of time keeping that secret, that's why I feel so relieved. Sometimes I feel alone, I feel that things are not the same with my friends and family. I grew up and everything changed. In December I said that I would never tell what was happening to me, that nobody would understand. I felt like a misfit. I didn't like my voice, it was weird.

My siblings don't know that I speak to you. I don't want them to know, let it be a secret."

X illuminates the clinic, bringing us closer to the way in which secrecy is presented as a way out of childhood, as a milestone in his pubertal subjective construction.

Conclusion

We consider the analytic clinic as a working space that is constructed in and from the analyst-patient duo and where the third party in absence is present.

What are we referring to? We allude to the creation of these multiple phantasmatic constructions that are gestated and arise out of the shared communication from unconscious to unconscious, between the participants of the field.

Therefore, it is worth conceiving the therapeutic relationship as an interplay where analyst and analysing create, in that analytical encounter, new text, new shared material.

Thus, in that encounter, a new meaning that brings them closer will emerge, it modifies and surpasses them both.

Interpretation will arise, fundamentally, from the exchange between the two subjectivities involved. Interpretation could then be expressed through the analytic word, but will only acquire value as such if it promotes a psychic change. The change might be displayed by a gestual, affective or verbal response from the patient.

Nowadays, as analysts, we cannot ignore the fact that the unconscious of both participants of the duo is traversed by external reality, by a historical and social moment that determines them.

Although we know that our work will take place in the transferential-countertransferential exchange that constitutes internal reality, the central object of psychoanalysis, it is absolutely necessary to recognise the traces of the epochal moment, those that promote changes in subjectivity.

Let us think of psychoanalysis as a constantly changing field. We extend an invitation to draw maps taking known routes, but with the courage to venture into new paths, to get lost in other territories that challenge us as analysts.

References

Aulagnier, P. 1980. *El derecho al secreto: Condición para poder pensar*. Sentido perdido. Editorial trieb, Buenos Aires.

Aulagnier, P. 2001. *La violencia de la interpretación*. Amorrtu editores, Buenos Aires.

Baranger, M. 1987. *El trauma psíquico infantil, de nosotros a Freud; Trauma puro, retroactividad y reconstrucción, Revista* de Psicoanálisis APA 64, no. 4.

Bauman, Z. 1999. *Modernidad líquida.* Editorial: Fondo de Cultura Económica. Buenos Aires.

Bleichmar, S. 2004. *Simbolizaciones de transición: una clínica abierta a lo real.* Docta. Año 2, no. 1.

Botella, S. and C. 2003. *La figurabilidad psíquica.* Amorrtu editores, Buenos Aires.

Freud, S. 1994. Obras Completas. Amorrortu editores, Buenos Aires.

Freud, S. 1994. *Cartas a Wilhelm Fliess Carta* 52. Obras Completas. Vol. 1, Amorrortu editores, Buenos Aires.

Freud, S. 1895/1950. *Proyecto de psicología,* Vol. 1 Amorrortu editores, Buenos Aires.

Freud, S. 1900/1994. *La interpretación de los sueños,* Vol. 5, Amorrortu editores, Buenos Aires.

Freud, S. 1914/1994. *Lo inconsciente.* Vol. 14, Amorrortu editores, Buenos Aires.

Freud, S. 1915/1994. *Pulsiones y destinos de pulsión.* Vol. 14, Amorrortu editores, Buenos Aires.

Freud, S. 1914/1994. *Introducción del Narcisismo.* Vol. 14, Amorrortu editores, Buenos Aires.

Freud, S. 1920/1994. *Más allá del Principio del Placer.* Vol. 18, Amorrortu editores, Buenos Aires.

Freud, S. 1923/1994. *El Yo y el Ello.* Vol. 18, Amorrortu editores, Buenos Aires.

Freud, S. 1930/1994. *El malestar en la cultura.* Tomo 21, Amorrortu editores, Buenos Aires.

Gallo, B. 1992. El analista y su inconsciente analizan. In: *Federación Psicoanalítica de América Latina. Malestar en el Psicoanálisis.* Montevideo, Federación Psicoanalítica de América Latina.

García Vázquez, S. 2010. *Trauma psíquico y método psicoanalítico. Revista Uruguaya de Psicoanálisis,* no. 100.

Green, A. 1999. *Narcisismo de vida, narcisismo de muerte.* Amorrortu editores, Buenos Aires.

Green, A. 2001. *De Locuras Privadas.* Amorrortu editores. Buenos Aires.

Marucco, N. 2015. *La persona y la función analítica ampliada. Revista de Psicoanálisis,* APA, 72, no. 2/3.

Paglini, J. 2011. *Clínica con niños Construyendo subjetividad.* Docta. *Revista de Psicoanálisis.* APC. 2012, no. 8

Paglini, J. 2015. Entre la Intimidad, Eros y Tánatos ¿Qué narcisismo? Docta. *Revista de Psicoanálisis.* APC, no. 12.

Paglini, J. 2018. *Tras este tiempo, vendrá otro... Subjetividades contemporáneas.* https://apcweb.com.ar/wp-content/uploads/2019/02/Tras-este-tiempo-vendra-otro.pdf.

Paglini, J. 2019. Lo infantil. Infancias posibles... *Revista de Psicoanálisis,* SPM, Año 1, no. 1, August 2021.

Paglini, J. et al. 2016. Regalo de quince: de lo intimidatorio a lo íntimo. *Revista de Psicoanálisis,* APA, 73, no. 4.

Real Academia Española. 2001. *Diccionario de la lengua española.* Madrid.

Viñoly Beceiro, A. M. 2006. Trabajando con las teorías. Una revisión de los ejes: tiempo-historia-estructura. In: *Tiempo, historia y estructura. Su impacto en el psicoanálisis contemporáneo*. Leticia Glocer Fiorini, compiladora. Ed. Lugar, Buenos Aires.

Winnicott, D. 1999. *Realidad y juego*. Ed. Gedisa. Buenos Aires.

Winnicott, D. 1981. *El proceso de maduración en el niño*. Editorial laia, Barcelona.

7 The Parental Unconscious

Trauma, Crypts, Fantasies and Failures

Vera Regina, J.R.M. Fonseca and Nilde Parada Franch

Introduction

"As psychoanalysts, we know that massive group trauma is transmitted intergenerationally (consciously) and transgenerationally (unconsciously...).

...Rage...which, in turn, fuels violence - functions as the psychological defense, par excellence, against unbearably painful feelings and memories... through our clinical work, psychoanalysts know that such traumatic feelings and memories tend to be discharged through action, for example in violence and aggression, as in war, rather than mastered through verbalization and the experiencing of unbearable feelings and memories in tolerable doses across time -which, very basically, describes the psychotherapeutic treatment of trauma".

(Ramzy, 2007, p. 308)

In many cultures, religion is linked to the cult of ancestors. ancestors would be our gods, as Meltzer (1983) pointed out, in his commentary on the religion of Klein's inner world: "Every person has to have a 'religion' in which his internal objects perform the function of Gods..." (1983, p. 38)

Following the thread of the generations, the parental unconscious will always be shaping styles, creating messages and evoking responses, which in turn will reverberate and compose the dyad's history, in what is expected to be a fluid and plastic mutual exchange.

But there are dyads in which such plasticity is replaced by rigid and unconscious mechanisms of transmission, particularly from experiences that have exceeded the processing capacity of the mind.

What is not processed has to be repeated, and so one sees stories repeating themselves and destinies being drawn.

Based on Bion's postulate that it is necessary to have two minds to think the most disturbing thoughts, Salberg (2015) states that parents might expel the traumatic unelaborated contents from their minds into the child's mind, in a process in search of containment, which can take three generations to resolve.

When referring to situations of unresolved mourning, Torok and Abrams (1984) used the term "crypt" to designate the mental place in which such

DOI: 10.4324/9781003246749-7

experiences are sheltered, isolated from psychic life. They denominate the offspring who will have to carry such a crypt as cryptophores (literally, those who carry the crypt), by means of an "endocryptical identification", in which the children "...become hosts to these unmourned deceased, the latter having developed a parasitical relationship to them... "cryptophores", constantly struggling with a "ghost effect", are the unconscious carriers, or carry in their unconscious, the crypts of their parents" (Demers, 1993, p. 32).

Dissociation would be the first step in all these processes of transgenerational transmission which might be identified in the various types of post-traumatic conditions, in which the experience of powerlessness, pain, fear and loss is so intense that the mind cannot bear it. In fact, several possibilities might result from this beginning, all depending on a certain degree of dissociation. We will mention a few:

- Identification with the aggressor, so well described by Fraiberg, Adelson and Shapiro (1975), in which vulnerability turns into hatred towards the next available and vulnerable object. This mechanism appears to underlie many cases of child abuse.
- Another possible destination is the unconscious transmission of the dissociated part to the children, in what Faimberg (1988, 1992) described as telescoping of generations. By telescoping she means the penetration of one lens into the other, over space / time (Trachtemberg et al., 2000).
- In other situations, what is transmitted is the depressive void, which can be directly translated by the child as his inability to be interesting to the mother, leading to the experience of futility and helplessness. This situation is masterfully described in the book *The Discomfort of Evening*, by Marieke Lucas Rijneveld, who won the International Booker Prize in 2020.

But how is trauma really transmitted? Would it be like a 'package', with all its content ready? Or would it be exactly the non-content, the absence of meaning that is transmitted? Or the presence of a ghost, as both Fraiberg and Torok and Abrams call it?

According to Kaës (1997), what is essentially transmitted are "...the configurations of psychic objects (affects, representations, fantasies), that is, objects plus their links, including the systems of object relations" (p. 14).

The film "Coco", directed by Lee Unkrich (Disney, 2017), masterfully illustrates the idea of transgenerational transmission of trauma in which transformations are possible only when someone (in this case, of the fourth generation) dared to seek the truth and unravel the mystery of post-traumatic resentment.

Let's now think in terms of development. Already in the prenatal period, the parental unconscious has a basic role in creating the space necessary for the development of the foetus's mind, opening up to the most primary processes that imply receptivity to the flow of the emotional contents of the rudimentary mind.

"If mother's mind is already inhabited by trauma (her own or her husband's) during gestation, her incapacity to differentiate will work as a shadow under which the fetus will be developing", (Cavalli, 2012, p. 610). It is a space that, to be receptive, needs to have both a containment limit and a neutral pressure, in order to allow the somato-psychic experiences of the foetus to flow. If there is a "positive pressure" or failure of a limiting membrane, the maternal contents can be pushed (or simply leaked[1]) into the foetus.

Finally, the transgenerational legacy in which narcissistic mental functioning prevails does not observe or respect the differences and subjectivities typical of the "other".

Clinical Examples

We[2] will describe a case that, in two different moments, evoked scenes in the analyst that she hypothesises were linked to the unconscious experiences of the parents.

Carol was an autistic six-year-old girl, in analysis with four sessions a week since the age of three. She practically did not develop language and ate compulsively, despite not being overweight. She had a marked preference for strings, using them in various ways, for example, tying them to the bars of the top shelf, trying to suspend herself on them.

First scene Analyst: "After countless sessions using the string I was sitting next to her on the sofa and had suddenly a clear view of an isolated foetus, with no connection to the mother's mind, having to entertain herself with the physicality of the umbilical cord. I recalled that Carol's mother became accidentally pregnant when living in a foreign country and experiencing both a depressive condition and an important eating disorder. I then wondered if having a baby in her womb could bring the feeling of being eaten inside, something she avoided by unconsciously cutting off contact with the foetus. The probable flaws in her own development and in her relationship with her primary objects perhaps did not provide her with sufficient mental space to shelter the mind of that foetus, with its unique characteristics".

Second scene "One day, trying to follow Carol's repetitive activities in a more 'fluid' way, I had an unexpected 'flash' of a village at war. I immediately remembered that Carol's father had spent his youth in war times in his country of origin. We had never talked about it before, which made me request to meet only with him in order to explore that topic. Nothing came, except factual reports, devoid of any engagement. I kept my hypothesis that the events were so disturbing and still tied him up so much in his current business that they could not be remembered in their real dimension of emotion".

After birth, in the initial stages of the dyadic relationship, the continuous process of communication and mutual modelling of the dyad is a vehicle par excellence for the transmission of the parental unconscious (Salberg, 2015). A young mother, coming from a family whose female lineage had several examples of histrionic theatrical behaviours, feared early on that her daughter would develop such flaws. When observing the mother-baby relationship, it was clear how all of the child's most expansive behaviours were repudiated, with those who showed greater regulation of emotional states and circumspection being better received. One can only imagine how much pressure such maternal expectations and attitudes had on the pair's communication and the child's development.

We want to bring two more clinical examples to illustrate the modes of penetration that the parents' unconscious can exercise in their children's mental lives.

The first case is from a supervision. A. was a five-year-old boy who came for analysis because he refused to go to school: he cried a lot, claiming he didn't want to be away from his mother. He also cried easily when his parents were more firm with him. A.'s mother had been sexually abused as a child and his father was a rather passive man.

To the analyst's surprise, A. revealed to be quite aggressive during the sessions, both with her and with his toys, especially with a doll. In addition, he often had highly sexualised behaviour, licking himself in the mirror with pleasure. One day, playing at being a demon that ate children, he said that some bad man beat him, and then he became "paranoid, crazy" (and he acted like he was really crazy): "The pervert entered through the window, and now he is here, with us". This sequence has been understood as the rebirth of the mother's repressed memory of abuse and the unconscious transmission of such registers to the child, turning him into a violent boy (or into a powerful phallus?). That would compensate the mother for her experience of helplessness and passivity when facing abuse.

The second case is of a teenager, Claudio, evaluated, owing to aggressive behaviours at home and at school, with a refusal to comply with basic rules. The parents reported that when he was two years old he was very violent towards his mother and grandmother, grabbing their hair and assaulting them, for no apparent reason. Over time, such behaviour improved, but the motivation for studying and socialising was very low. During the assessment, the father, whom we will call Bruno, told the analyst about his own childhood, living with his grandmother in an extremely violent neighbourhood, as his own mother had left him and fled with a "bank robber". In order to survive, he also became violent, to the point of being nicknamed "the madman"; then he was helped by relatives and was able to graduate from university, get married, and have two children, becoming a very "peaceful" person. During the psychoanalytic observation, Claudio seemed quite detached, showing scarce motivation or personal ambition. He told the analyst how he spent his days locked in his room playing video games. An inner emptiness and a sense that nothing was meaningful were evident.

In the final conversation with the parents, Bruno confessed to the analyst that both his son and he were "healed" by spiritualism: one night, in Claudio's cradle, he saw an evil spirit trying to steal his baby son. He firmly opposed this force, prayed aloud for a long time, and got the spirit to leave. Such an "interpretation" was, in the analyst's view, an attempt to give some meaning to the violence suffered during childhood, but it was clear how these unprocessed experiences demanded to be relived in the next generations, as a violent spirit/ghost that left no space for the development of a proper and alive self for Claudio.

We now pose a technical question: What does the analyst interpret from her reverie? What can she 'see' of the unrepresented events from other generations dwelling in the patient's internal world? Cavalli (2012) states that the analyst will not do a direct translation, but rather should facilitate the creation of space and language to accept death, loss, trauma, keeping hope alive and allowing continuity for the next generations, with its potential to create new paths and experiences. Sometimes, however, a real historical reconstruction ends up being carried out.

The Biological Perspective

Finally, we want to present some data from research done in the field of biology on intergenerational transmission of traumas, in which the "nurture" of one generation can become the "nature" of the other (Yehuda and Lehrner, 2018). Until a few decades ago, such ideas were viewed with scepticism by the traditional scientific community. But clinical evidence eventually prevailed, revealing several cases in which survivors of genocide and war, that were able to function within normal limits, had children and grandchildren with severe psychiatric conditions. Animal studies also brought surprising data, which were later corroborated and/or expanded in the subsequent multiple investigations of human cases. The most prevalent idea is that the effects of trauma for a generation are transmitted through epigenetic, non-genomic mechanisms (that is, without changing the DNA sequence). Epigenetic refers to the fact that events and characteristics of the environment prevent the expression of some genes, "turning them off" through a methylation process, which impairs their transcription. Another means of transmitting the effects of trauma would be the foetus-placental interactions, in which hormonal changes occurring in stressful situations impact the regulatory structures of the foetus itself, an effect that remains after birth. It has also been found, for example, that hunger and severe stress during pregnancy can affect up to the third generation, with different results depending on the time of pregnancy and the sex of the foetus (for example, prenatal stress in humans has been associated with changes in daytime cortisol secretion in boys, but not in girls). The effects of trauma preceding conception can also be transmitted through changes in the gametes themselves, whether maternal or paternal, also with different potential effects.

But the most important point of such research for psychoanalysis is that:

> "...the principle of epigenetic plasticity implies that changes to the epigenome might reset when the environmental insults are no longer present, or when we have changed sufficiently to address environmental challenges in a new way. It is the ability to flexibly respond to environmental stimuli that is fundamentally adaptive and the basis of human resilience".
>
> (Yehuda and Lehrner, 2018, p. 253)

Therefore, being unconscious (even somatic), parental factors will need the presence of another mind to be transformed, making clear the importance of analytical work.

Notes

1 See Felton (apud Rosenfeld, 1987).
2 The clinical examples come from the clinic of one of the authors.

References

Abraham, N. and Torok, M. 1984. "The Lost Object—Me": Notes on Identification within the Crypt. *Psychoanal. Inq.*, 4(2): 221–242.

Cavalli, A. 2012. Transgenerational Transmission of Indigestible Facts: From Trauma, Deadly Ghosts and Mental Voids to Meaning-Making Interpretations. *J. Anal. Psychol.*, 57(5): 597–614.

Demers, L.A. 1993. Intergenerational Grief: Who's Mourning Whom?. *Canadian J. Psychoanal.*, 1(1): 27–40.

Faimberg, H. 1988. The Telescoping of Generations: Genealogy of Certain Identifications. *Contemp. Psychoanal.*, 24: 99–117.

Faimberg, H. 1992. A la escucha del telescopaje de generaciones: pertinencia psicoanalitica del concepto. *Rev. Psicoanál. Asoc. Psico.* 15: 9–24.

Fraiberg, S., Adelson, E. and Shapiro, V. 1975. Ghosts in the Nursery: A Psychoanalytic Approach to the Problems of Impaired Infant-Mother Relationships. *Journal of the American Academy of Child Psychiatry*, Vol. 14, no. 3: 387–421.

Kaës, R. 1977. *Dispositivos psicoanaliticos y emergenciais de lo geracional*. In: Lo geracional. Buenos Aires: Amorrortu, 1977, p. 14.

Meltzer, D. 1983. *Dream-Life: A Re-Examination of the Psychoanalytic Theory and Technique*. London: Karnac Books.

Ramzy, N. 2007. Intergenerational and Transgenerational Transmission of Hatred and Violence: Some Psychoanalytic Comments for the Prevention and Amelioration of Hatred and Violence in the Palestinian-Israeli Conflict. *Int. J. Appl. Psychoanal. Stud.*, 4(3): 308–309.

Rosenfeld, H. 1987. Projective Identification in Clinical Practice. In: *Impasse and Interpretation: Therapeutic and anti-therapeutic factors in the psychoanalytic treatment of psychotic, borderline, and neurotic patients. New Library of Psychoanalysis.* London: Tavistock.

Salberg, J. 2015. The Texture of Traumatic Attachment: Presence and Ghostly Absence in Transgenerational Transmission. *Psychoanal Q.,* 84(1): 21–46.

Trachtenberg, A.R. et al. 2000. Entrevista com Haydée Faimberg (Interview with Haydée Faimberg). *Revista Psicanálise, Sociedade Brasileira Psicanalítica de Porto Alegre.* Vol. 2. no. 1: 249–266.

Tratchenberg, A.R. et al. 2013. *Transgeracionalidade – de escravo a herdeiro: um destino entre gerações.* Porto Alegre: Sulina.

Yehuda, R. and Lehrner, A. 2018. Intergenerational transmission of trauma effects: putative role of epigenetic mechanisms. *World Psychiatry.* 17(3): 243–257. doi:10.1002/wps.20568.

8 Remembering and Working Through the Trauma of Paternal Loss and Maternal Postpartum Depression

The Case of Sam

There are theoretical debate and questions what constitutes trauma and what is the external reality versus internal conflicts influencing the experience of trauma. While most agree with the following definition of trauma, as "any experience which calls up distressing affect such as those of fright, anxiety, shame, physical pain". There are also disagreements in our field, and disputes about the role of external reality versus internal conflicts continue to appear in the psychoanalytic literature.

The study of hysteria has paved the way for the growth of psychoanalytic theory ever since Breuer and Freud made an effort to sort out its clinical presentation in the mid-1890s. Dissociative processes fuel the engine that drives hysteria along peculiarly predictable paths. The vertical split represents a description of a dissociative organisation of mind. A multiple self-state model of mind sits at the core of self-psychology.

The notion of trauma also emerged in all its importance in Ferenczi's work. Subsequent papers by Freud and after the Second World War by post-Freudians such as Winnicott, Balint, Klein, Heimann, Fairbairn, Bion, Ogden, and others have become our travelling companions. With reference to scattered remarks in Ferenczi's (1932) *Clinical Diary* and in some of his less known works, this account reconstructs the dramatic process of the analysis of Ferenczi's highly important patient, his colleague "R.N." (Elizabeth Severn). It shows how much we can learn from these historical documents and from the experience that underlies them. Comments, remarks and questions take us to the very heart of Ferenczi's psychoanalytical thinking. They might well provide a stimulus for thinking again about some important topics that have to do with psychoanalysis as it is practiced in contemporary society and the problems of human relationships and emotions in general.

From point of view of Fonagy's the disrupt of mentalisation is the result of early traumatic experience. The use of the term *trauma* in psychoanalytic theory suggests that the key element for a theory of pathogenesis and mental functioning is not the either/or of external versus internal causation or trauma versus drive. Rather, it is an understanding of whether, or to what extent, the raw data of existential experience is or is not transformed into *psychological* experience. From this perspective, trauma is

DOI: 10.4324/9781003246749-8

whatever outstrips and disrupts the psyche's capacity for representation or mentalisation. Absent the potential for mental representation, these events and phenomena are historical only from an external, third-person perspective. Until they are mentalised, they remain locked within a historical, repetitive process as potentials for action, somatisation and projection.

In cases of extreme childhood trauma associated with abuse and neglect, one's sense of self is seriously compromised. Attachment patterns, symptoms, defensive operations, and character formation will differ depending upon the level of interference and impingement. When repeated trauma occurs in early childhood, the dissociative response might become the first line of defence for the person to rely upon. In its most severe form, patients are diagnosed with dissociative identity disorder (DID). The restoration of a cohesive sense of self from the parts that are dissociated, and fragmented self is the aim of therapy.

Sugarman (2003) offers a useful perspective. He combines both approaches, favouring neither, recognising the capacity of the brain to filter, organise and structure information at different levels. He recognises, as do others Busch (2005), that traumatic experiences and memories also become part of one's internal conflicts in reaction to which an entire venue of defences develop and operate quite unconsciously, such as the psychological process of not wanting to know the trauma.

Van der Kolk, McFarlane and Weisaeth (1996) have also expanded the deepening of our understanding of traumatic experiences and how they are stored in the brain.

The notion that traumatic memories are encoded differently in the brain has both implications for recall during treatment as well as the technical considerations in working with traumatised children.

Within the context of play technique, the repetitive re-enactment of games (related to traumatic events) suggests the possibility that children might face re-traumatisation within the clinical situation. Traumatic memories coded in a different part of brain utilise memory processes that are not readily available for verbal expression.

Lenore Terr uses the distinction between procedural (implicit) versus declarative (explicit) memory to argue for technical interventions that do not privilege verbal expression as a marker of insight and therapeutic gain. They emphasise the emotional interaction between the child and the analyst as the focal point of the therapeutic action. The re-experience of procedural memories in the analytical relationship is a crucial aspect of the analytical process.

However, there are others who believe that inability of a patient to put words could be the evidence of an underlying defence and resistance, such as Bohleber. The role of interpretation in facilitating self-reflection and thinking are emphasised. Yet there are other psychoanalysts like Gaensbauer and Bauer and Wewerka who suggest that traumatic memories are not markedly different from other memory processes, and preverbal traumas are remembered both procedurally and declaratively. With therapeutic relationship at the centre of our work, the questions regarding the transformative power of play itself can then be raised. The importance of play in mastering trauma and promoting self- reflection has been highlighted by more recent contemporary child analysts. Sugarman (2008) writes, "Language is less often a useful vehicle for promoting insight than behavioural enactments and assisting children in developing a narrative in their play helps them consider multiple relationship paradigm's articulate affect states, distinguishing different emotions, and learning the difference between acting on and speaking about feelings".

While traumatised children use play to cope with stress using displacement, identifications with aggressor, turning passive into active, and denials they also benefit from when their analysts facilitate their imaginary play. Conscious recall of traumatic memories is not always possible with young children, and sometimes self-reflective capacities, indicative of mentalising processes, could be inhibited or denied, avoiding painful affects.

Nonverbal communication, at both conscious and unconscious levels, can be portrayed as a type of "body language," a communication between the psychic bodies of patient and therapist. In this article, the author provides several examples of this communication process in the context of a psychoanalytic treatment with a patient who has a history of trauma resulting in frequent dissociative states. Motoric actions (drawing), somatosensory symptoms, and intense affect states represent the media through which she "informs" the analyst of her painful experiences. The analyst's surrender to countertransference states, such as deadness, constitutes the beginning of attunement to the patient's body communications. In one particularly unusual symptom of dissociation, the patient exhibits physical abilities that she is incapable of in more integrated states. An attempt is made to understand this event from a Phenom-enological and neurobiological perspective. Using an information-processing model, the patient's sub symbolic information might be converted to the verbal symbolic via the analyst's use of evoked images.

Sugarman (2003) noted, "The ability to play and to fantasize freely becomes a guidepost or sign of analytic progress and mental health in the child" (p. 343).

Working through play and encouraging the development of a narrative becomes a necessary step to help these children access their internal anxieties and wishes over time.

The case I present illustrate the repetitive nature of traumatic play and how the analyst function as observer and participant, and how the analyst facilitates affect regulation, frustration tolerance, and acquisition of skills by mutual interactive play.

My case concerns a young boy who seemed to have a great difficulty in knowing about his object loss, both in external reality and in his internal world.

Sam, a five-year-old boy was referred by his paediatrician to me for analytical treatment, because of his presenting symptom of sensory motor integration problem and the regressive symptoms after the recent loss of his father to leukaemia.

He showed regressive behaviour like singing in singsong voice, chewing his blanket and sucking his thumb, after he was separated from his parents at age four in order to live with his paternal aunt during his father's course of treatment.

Sam had a sister who was two-and-a-half years older than him. After his father was diagnosed with lymphoma, he went through several rounds of chemotherapy. His mother suffered from postpartum depression after Sam was born.

The attachment between mother and son was a mixture of insecure/anxious/avoidant type, which was described poignantly by his mother through her statement about Sam: "I did not care taking care of him I was so burdened with my own depression that I wished he would turn into a three-year-old who could tell me what he wanted, not an infant! I was depressed when he was born. What could I have done? There was no energy to deal with him, when I had no energy left to handle myself, him and my daughter!"

He was described as a colicky baby who could not be soothed. Mother felt frustrated with him and wished she never had him.

The real physical separation from his mother occurred when Sam was a toddler, because his father's health deteriorated. He became bed ridden at home and was admitted to the hospital shortly after that. Sam's mother could not take care of him, yet she had to be present at her husband's bedside in the hospital. The entire course of father's diagnosis, treatment and finally at the end his traumatic death lasted for two years.

His father's absence was unpredictable because of the nature of his illness. He would return home for few weeks and then suddenly he had to be admitted to the hospital.

His disappearance was unpredictable. Sam did not know when he would return home. He lived with his paternal aunt for almost a year, and occasionally visited his father in the hospital. The aunt had her own two school age kids to take care of and Sam lived with his aunt and cousin while his sister lived with his mother.

His mother reported that she could not remember if she told him in words that his father died in the hospital. One day, when he asked to see his father, he was told he could not see him because he was gone to be in heaven.

The memory of his father's death was unavailable in the verbal realm, and it was only expressed later in his analysis. The way in which it appeared was in some form of a *belief* regarding him "someday" coming back to visit Sam or Sam would go to visit his father in the heaven.

He resorted to Peek-a-Boo play repeatedly with me during the beginning phase of his analysis.

During this period, Sam wanted to know if I could see him every day. I told him that he wanted to remember me by coming to see me every day and not to forget how I looked. I also told him, "You want to know whether I remembered you when I do not see you over the weekend" Later, I added to my interpretation that it must have been hard for him not knowing where his father was and not remembering his face. He nodded and said, "I thought someday, he would come home!"

He was quiet and seemed to be listening intently. I also added that even though people do not see each other, some still can remember the person. "When your mother had to be with your father in the hospital, you were not sure if she remembered you when she could not see you. Now with me, you want to make sure we both remember each other at all times".

There was another fantasy about father and son reunion that had to do with him taking a train or plane to visit his dad in "heaven". He debated if he should take a train or plane and asked my opinion. According to his mother it was his religious paternal grandmother who planted the idea of "heaven" in his mind. These fantasies were prominent at the beginning of his first year of treatment.

Our initial interactions, were characterised with his earlier infantile developmental stage, gaze-turn-taking which was matched with my voice intonation when I called him by his name. This resembled to me an earlier mother-infant mode of communication. These moments were punctuated with a different kind of interaction that were belonged to a somewhat higher level of development with prominent use of his verbal precocity to name his feelings followed with periods characterised with absence of words, thoughts and feeling state. His verbal precocity was noteworthy and yet manifested itself with alternated period of long silences with blank face. As if he was in another space, disconnected from me.

His precocious selective verbal ability together with areas of more primitive loss of connection with parental objects especially with maternal object created an unusual patchwork in his internal psychic landscape.

Later, as his analysis moved forward, he became fascinated with the sand tray in the playroom of my office. Making animals disappear and again making them gleefully reappear and making them rise from their burial spots, which was repetitious and had symbolic tone and flavor and to it.

Here, I observed his transition from a non-verbal to symbolic state where he used displacement and dealt with inner fantasies and conflicts. He used this game numerous times repeatedly, to bridge the transition from our missed sessions to seeing each other in his appointed sessions. His experience marked his active killing off the link where the analytic object was lost and followed by "reviving the broken contact with me".

I also made additional containing gestures on my own part by making a calendar and showing him the days, we would see each other. At the end of each session, he wanted to leave his drawing with me, but wanted also to keep a copy for himself.

This was another gesture to make sure he restored his link with me between the sessions. In the analytic process, the trauma of paternal object loss was re-evoked by the dynamic of loss between the two of us i.e., him as a child and me as his analyst/developmental parents. There were aspects of trusting encounters, which gradually was formed within the reliability of a safe holding analytic space, and his experience of me as a safe object. The analytic setting offered a potential *space* where transference relationship developed further despite of an early object loss.

Trauma of paternal object loss repeatedly played out between us. He was super-sensitive about my absences during weekends or my vacation break. He imagined I was going away on the other side of the earth like his father who disappeared and turned into ashes. His ashes were actually scattered in the ocean. His mother quite anxiously dealt with her grief by taking her two children on a boat to scatter his ashes in the river without any prior warning. I found out afterward, that one day she woke up and decided to take a trip to the coastal region near where they lived to scatter his ashes without preparing her children in advance rather on an impulse without planning.

Sam talked about it without showing any feeling, with a flat affect. It was as if he and his sister were given a job to spread one fistful of his father's ashes onto the ocean. They did it dutifully without any word exchange and rather mechanically.

Sam brought his drawings to show me on a regular and frequent basis, which showed a repeated act of displaying a self-representation in the form of fragmented parts of self which was laced with a clear evidence of absence of affect. The original traumatic experience of seeing his father for an extended period with swollen and disfigured face and body on the hospital bed was also represented in his drawings only at a later stage of his analysis. He showed me how he remembered his paternal grandmother's words by repeating them. He told me that his grandmother told him over and over that if he were a good boy, he would see his father in the heaven and if he were naughty, he would go to Hell.

He feared that he would be the latter and would go to Hell. He asked me one day if I knew where Hell was. Then, he told me that all he knew about was the fact that he was convinced that it must have been a terrible "black hole". He feared that he would fall in the hole, and no one could ever find him.

He enacted a violent fighting, with scenes of shooting and knifing during a playful exchange between the two of us. He was afraid that we both would end up dying a terrible death. These behaviours looked like the somatic form of his dissociation, which was consistent with signs and symptoms of posttraumatic syndrome.

Later, as our work continued close to the end of the second year of his analysis, he recovered a memory of his father on his hospital bed. He saw his father's face *disfigured, swollen,* looking *disgusting and scary* on the hospital bed hooked up to tubes. He was unsure if the man was his father that he had always known. His mother assured him that his father loved him and his sister, even though he could not say it himself in words. He was unable to think about his father as a dead person.

His unresolved feelings and traumatic experience of his massive loss made him to be prone to have dissociative symptoms. Sam's insecure, anxious attachment to his mother was directly linked to his absent and mis-attuned mother.

Winnicott's notion of splitting and dissociation fits with Shane's case.

Carlson's study in 1998 identified a direct association between dissociated symptoms at 17 years and a disorganised attachment at 12 to 18 months, while Liotti linked dissociative symptoms to parental experience of loss. She assesses whether the patients' absence of thought and unrepresented moments are a feature of repression or dissociation. She shows how this awareness shaped her theoretical understanding and subsequent intervention strategies better suited to disrupted associative mental capacities.

My work with his mother in the *parent-work* of the treatment was extremely important and instrumental, since I could parent his mother who was traumatised by losing her husband to cancer. I also helped her to create boundary between herself and her son rather treating him as an extension of her.

My consistent presence and capacity to survive Sam's enactment, evocations of his traumatic past, my ability to contain his aggressive attacks and communications in our play as well as my work with his mother and maternal grandparents with whom he has been living after his father's death were important focus at the centre of my analytic work. This resulted the progression of the analytical process which led to his analytical gains.

I had to work through my counter-transference feelings, which oscillated from a wide range of hopefulness, despair and my rescuer fantasy. I had to metabolise my own unbearable feelings especially when I worked with his mother in parent work.

The parent-work was instrumental, since I knew that I had to parent his mother by being an optimal container for her un-metabolised traumatic experience earlier in her life when he lost her brother to a severe mental illness, and her most recent loss of her husband to the cancer. It was also helpful to his mother to learn how to establish boundary between herself and her son. She realised that she was being permissive out of sense of guilt and not recognising her parental authority by claiming to be a generation separate from her son, rather obliterating the generational boundary by descending to his.

In my analytical work with Sam, I provided him a transitional space to move upward in his development. The trust got established which gradually formed within the reliability of a safe holding space.

In the back of my mind with my theoretical frame, I found Winnicott's idea very helpful, his idea of the development of play that depends on the creation and building of trust.

Freud's reality principle, consciousness of impression sense, attention, memory, judgment, and thought were compromised because of the trauma Shane had to endure. The world brought him a catastrophe and his internal connections to his object relation were smashed. His frustration intolerance was the provocation and trigger for his regressive behaviour as well as his self-destructive behaviour.

The question I keep asking myself has to do as to whether his lack of attachment bonding and disconnectedness to his maternal object representation caused him to develop a dissociative state of mind along with developmental regression. In his case, there has been a narcissistic injury. His narcissism was a negative reaction to connection to his objects, owing to his dual object losses.

I also wondered whether part of this regression was linked to the nature of the experiences in the psychic register that were pre-verbal. My effort to verbalise his affect initially was fruitless until I was able to understand his active killing off the object through his play and reviving the disconnected contact with his object by a repetitious play of making objects disappear and reappear.

I know there would be a future need for him to engage in further remaining analytical works that ought to continue in future work with him.

There follows an excerpt from his analytical process.

1 Excerpt of one of the sessions in his second year of analysis

During this hour, Shane showed up accompanied with his grandfather. He looked happy to see me. He brought with him his drawing. He drew many circles on top of each other, and under the heap of all the circles, there is one circle hidden somewhere very deep. He said that is him (his face with nothing on it and an empty circle) laying under several other circles.

He said: "I am trying to hide myself and when I do it, no one will ever find me, then that is when I feels lonely!" Then he went on to tell me "When you find me behind the curtain (Peek-a-Boo) I am happy that you find me".

A: I said: "When no one is around to find you, you feel lonely, and you are not sure if I remember you when you do not see me".

At this point, he moves his right hand to the front of his pants and slid it inside his pants. He leaves it there. He looks quiet and looked like he is holding on to his penis and being was being silent. After a brief pause, he said "see Dr. Mann, I don't want my penis to hop away! I don't want to explode when I go pee pee!"

A: "You just told me how you feel lonely when no one notices you or finds you. You want to show me your feelings through the drawing you brought today. Now, you want to show me how you are both scared of being alone and excited! Especially those times that you go to pee."

Shane: "See, I want to see if it is still there! Hey penis, are you there?" .... "Nobody will blow my penis up! A bunch of pee will come around. When my bladder is full, then it gets squeezed out, it makes me excited!"

A: "By touching it, you make sure *it* is there and *it* is part of you. You want to keep it there with your hand holding it tight; this way, it will not leave you on its own without you knowing".

Shane: "sometimes my penis gets excited and makes me jump around and scream".

A: "It is not easy to figure out your feelings when it happens".

2 Excerpt from a recent session

During this hour, Shane showed up looking tired and not his usual excited self.

Shane: "I could not fall sleep last night! My mom was O.K. with it. mom was happy for me to go and draw on a piece of paper. I used the CAPS! I wanted to get my anger out. That is why I use the CAPS! I also used a chewy toy to chew on, but not the squeeze ball. One of my teachers in Cameron Park (this is the period the two children lived with paternal aunt away from their parents because of father's illness) would give me a prize when I did a good job. Then, we moved here to live with my grandparents".

A: "You had to move a few times when you father was ill! You had to leave people you knew behind and come to a new school".

Shane: "See, I moved here when I was five. I lost my Dad two years ago! I remember I could not hear my mom whenever she talked to me".

A: "Those were very tough time for you and, you were trying hard to figure things out! Lot of feelings had to get sorted out and getting to know new people in your life. When I came to live with my grandparents, I talked to Pappi (his grandfather). They had rabies, because it is a type of disease that raccoon, cats and dead animals have. They have something, which is a type of disease you can go to the hospital. You can have it or not. I don't think all people have it. Sometimes animals get disease on them, which cause rabies!"

A: "It seems to me you are thinking whole lot about how what animals get ill and how people get ill".

Shane: "Yeah, ... I don't know why!"

"I know, there is a dead rat in my street. What happens if you touch a dead rat that has rabies? Do I get it?"

"I don't think I touched it though".

After a short pause, he continued, "My mom lifted me up to see "my Dad in his coffin". He was dressed fancy in his coffin. I don't ever cry when someone dies. He looked regular! He had a fancy shirt He was laying in his casket with his hands crossed. His eyes closed and no breathing at all. He was still! There was a tie around his neck. Then he got turned into ashes".

A: "It is hard for you to understand how he got turned into ashes next thing you knew. It must have been confusing".

Shane: "It is too extreme for my age to know how someone turns into ashes. You see, my Dad's parents are catholic. Maybe I can ask my grandma (maternal grand ma). I can also ask her when I go to see my dad if he is there waiting for me in heaven".

After a few seconds, he asked, "Have you been to heaven? I bet you did. It is because you are a good doctor!"

Discussion

In our clinical practice, we must deal with traumatic events characterised by the fact that *something that should have happened did not happen* and the subject is left lacking that work of affective significance necessary to subjectivation and to feeling that he and his own feelings are "real" (in the sense of Winnicott's *realness*). In Shane case, the death of his father happened and it was not unreal, but fact. These situations are based on rigid and repetitive past *relational sequences* characterised by such a deficit in *mirroring* or *rêverie* that the individual's subjectivity is wounded and his autonomous psychic existence is damaged. These sequences take shape in the mind as experiences that, by virtue of the damage inflicted on the representative faculty, belong to the sphere of the not named and the not symbolised.

The therapeutic encounter with patients who are seriously traumatised has led psychoanalytic research to focus its attention on the importance of the construction and/or reconstruction of the mind's *symbolic capacity*. Concerning this point, numerous authors, concur that today the analyst's principal task is to restore the thought functions necessary for becoming capable of dealing with previously unbearable and un-representable psychic suffering: a necessarily preliminary work to that on *splitting* or *repression*.

This view of the analytic process has its roots in the Bionian concept of *containment*. By 1958 Bion had already intuited that if the patient was denied the opportunity for a normal use of projective identification this provoked serious problems: with such a denial, the analyst in fact destroyed an extremely important bond. In introducing the concepts of *containment* and *negative capability*, Bion added functions to the analyst's tools that were not interpretative but participative, making the analytic situation more interpersonal.

Regarding this point, Grotstein recently described Bion as *one of the founders of inter-subjectivity* and emphasised the clinical meaningfulness of Bion's concept of *becoming*, which denotes the analyst's capacity to work in such a way that his own unconscious *resonates with that of the patient's*, getting "into the skin" of the analysand while remaining, at the same time, in his own. In other words, for Grotstein *the analyst must temporarily become the analysand*.

In these situations, "interpreting" becomes a crucial element in the analysis, not so much in the traditional sense of giving interpretations, but rather in the sense of *personifying*—for long periods and unknowingly—specific characters and roles from the patient's history and internal world. This aspect (explored by Melanie Klein in "Personification in the play of children" of 1929) is something which, with Franco Borgogno, we have focused on in various works, emphasising how essential it is for the analyst to "lend" his emotional and symbolic functions, *experimenting emotions in search of an author* for however long is necessary, so that the patient will eventually be able to find them within himself.

In fact, the *characters* that patients *unconsciously come to play and interpret through the acting out* that is intrinsic to repetition are those aspects of themselves that they are unable to accept as theirs and to show to the world with ease: those parts of the self that do not seem able to meet the other in a satisfactory manner. Playing offers an approach to this problematic part of one's personality: you can be something and then immediately afterwards repudiate it; playing allows one to encounter unrecognised and delegitimised aspects of the self by controlling the ways and times. In this sense analysis would seem to have been conceived deliberately for playing: the analyst offers himself as a transitional object and can be *used as the other character* necessary for unknowingly representing the individual drama that is acted out in the transference.

From this standpoint, it becomes essential to view the setting, in line with Winnicott, not as an inert space but as an empathic environment capable of restoring to the analysand his experiences "understood", in such a way that they can be further worked through mentally by the patient himself with the help of the analyst.

Such a setting takes the form of a "three-dimensional", transitional, playful space; a *potential space* for growth in which all the various components—narrative and symbolic, but also pre-symbolic and acted—of the transference relationship can develop and so allow the individual who has never managed to become himself to construct the meanings of his own subjective experience. Precisely in this potential space, the *serious game* that is analysis takes place: it is an *intermediate space* shared by the analyst and the patient in which creative transformations are produced. In fact, psychotherapy takes place in the overlap of two areas of playing, that of the patient and that of the therapist. So psychotherapy has to do with two people playing together. The "corollary" of this is that where playing is not possible then the work done by the therapist is directed towards bringing the patient from a state of not being able to play into a state of being able to play.

An analysis conceived in this way cannot be carried out by an ideally "neutral" analyst, or, better, *neutrality* has to be thought of as an uninterrupted activity between identification and dis-identification: in order to preserve it the analyst will always have to resort to his capacity for being identified with the patient and yet also quite distinct.

The transformative potential of analysis lies in the dialectic participation of the analyst in a role now of "old" object now of "new" object: for the analysis to be truly mutative, the therapist must, in fact, be capable of activating the patient's pre-existing fears and hopes. However, at the same time, something new and unexpected must happen within the relationship that can lead to a gradual remodelling of his internal object representations through a well-calibrated balance between interpretation and containment as therapeutic factors, in dialectic tension with each other.

References

American Psychiatric Association. 1994. *The diagnostic and statistical manual of mental disorders, 4th ed. (DSM-IV)*, Washington, DC: American Psychoanalytic Press.

Bass, G. 2002. Something is happening here: Thoughts and clinical material regarding multiplicity, gender and touch in a psychoanalytic treatment. *Psychoanalytic Dialogues*, 12: 809–826.

Bowlby, J. 1969. *Attachment and loss: Volume I, attachment*, New York, NY: Basic Books.

Brenner, I. 2001. *Dissociation of trauma: Theory, phenomenology, and technique*, Madison, CT: International Universities Press.

Brenner, I. 1994. The dissociative character: A reconsideration of "multiple personality". *Journal of the American Psychoanalytic Association*, 42: 819–846.

Brenner, I. 2001. *Dissociation of trauma: Theory, phenomenology, and technique*, Madison, CT: International Universities Press.

Bromberg, P. 1998. *Standing in the spaces: Essays on clinical process trauma & dissociation*, Hillsdale, NJ: Analytic Press.

Bromberg, P. 1998. *Standing in the spaces: Essays on clinical process trauma & dissociation*, Hillsdale, NJ: Analytic Press.

Davies, J. and Frawley, M.G. 1994. *Treating the adult survivor of childhood abuse: A psychoanalytic perspective*, New York, NY: Basic Books.

Farber, S. 2008. Dissociation, traumatic attachment, and self-harm: eating disorders and self-mutilation. *Clinical Social Work Journal*, 36: 63–72.

Fonagy, P. 2001. *Attachment theory and psychoanalysis*, New York, NY: Other Press.

Gold, S.N. 2000. *Not trauma alone: Therapy for childhood survivors in family and social context*, Philadelphia, PA: Brunner/Routledge.

Gold, S.N. 2000. *Not trauma alone: Therapy for childhood survivors in family and social context*, Philadelphia, PA: Brunner/Routledge.

Howell, E. 2005. *The dissociative mind*, Hillsdale, NJ: Analytic Press.

Josephs, L. 1995. *Balancing empathy and interpretation: Rational character analysis*, Northvale, NJ: Aronson.

Kluft, R. 1982. Varieties of hypnotic interventions in the treatment of multiple personality. *American Journal of Clinical Hypnosis*, 26: 73–83.

Kluft, R. 1993. *Clinical approaches to the integration of personalities: Clinical perspectives on multiple personality disorder*, Washington, DC: American Psychiatric Press.

Loewenstein, R. and Ross, D. 1992. Multiple personality and psychoanalysis: An introduction. *Psychoanalytic Inquiry*, 12: 3–48.

Loewenstein, R. and Ross, D. 1992. Multiple personality and psychoanalysis: An introduction. *Psychoanalytic Inquiry*, 12: 3–48.

Novick, J. and Novick, K.K. 1996. *Fearful symmetry: The development and treatment of sadomasochism*, Northvale, NJ: Aronson.

Novick, J. and Novick, K.K. 2000. Love in the therapeutic alliance. *Journal of the American Psychoanalytic Association*, 48: 189–218.

Putnam, F. 1989. *Diagnosis and treatment of multiple personality disorder*. New York, NY: Guilford.

Putnam, F. 1992. Dissociation: Are alter personalities fragments or figments?*Psychoanalytic Inquiry*, 12: 95–111.

Schore, A. 2003. *"Affect dysregulation and disorders of the self"*. New York, NY: W.W. Norton & Company.

Schwartz, H.L. 1994. From dissociation to negotiation: A relational psychoanalytic perspective on multiple personality disorder. *Psychoanalytic Psychology*, 11: 189–231.

Steinbeck, J. 1939. *The Grapes of Wrath*, New York, NY: Viking.

Winnicott, D.W. 1960. *The maturational processes and the facilitating environment*, Madison, CT: International Universities Press.

Winnicott, 1960. *Healthy development is predicated upon a "good-enough" environment*. Madison, CT: International Universities Press.

Winnicott, D.W. 1960. *The maturational processes and the facilitating environment*, Madison, CT: International Universities Press.

9   Notes on Breakdown in Child Development: Misconceptions and Disorientations

Emanuela Quagliata

Introduction

In this paper I shall first refer to those theories which I have found most useful when considering my clinical experience with patients, children and adolescents, who come for analysis when a breakdown in their development occurs. The parents state that up to that moment their son or daughter has not shown any particular problem; they often describe them as autonomous children and not very demanding. However, following an apparently insignificant event, they inexplicably seem to lose contact with reality: they show deep and intense anxieties in the form of emotional and cognitive disorganisation: a sudden breakdown in their development.

Since the very beginning, psychoanalysis has turned its attention to the earliest moments of a child's life, and when reflecting on the origin of neuroses, Freud wrote to his friend Fliess: "Everything is leading me towards focusing on the earliest stages of life, up to the third year" (Freud, 1897).

Melanie Klein was convinced of the existence of an early rudimentary ego and some degree of innate object-relatedness from birth. Infant research and the neurosciences seem to agree with this hypothesis, according to which babies have competence and readiness for engagement - i.e they are born equipped to interact with others - and more recent studies demonstrate that from the prenatal phase, the foetus might be aware of its interaction with the uterine environment (Stern, 1985; Trevarthen, 1979; Alhanati, 2002; Mancia, 1981).

Klein also reasoned that "the young infant feels unconsciously every discomfort as though it were inflicted on him by hostile forces. If comfort is given to him soon—in particular warmth, the loving way he is held, and the gratification of being fed—this gives rise to happier emotions [...] My hypothesis is that the infant has an innate unconscious awareness of the existence of the mother" (1959, p. 248).

Bion (1962a, 1962b) thought that the infant is incapable of making use of the chaotic sensory data (*beta elements*) and that this incapacity manifests itself in the form of distress and anxiety which the child must release,

DOI: 10.4324/9781003246749-9

projecting them into the mother. He extends Klein's concept of projective identification to include the fundamental role it plays in the primitive communication and interactions between mother and baby (Bion, 1962a, 1962b). Therefore, in these exchanges, the mother remains the mother and the child remains the child. The child relies on her so that his discomfort is taken in, thought about and transformed into elements that can be made thinkable (*alpha elements*). Experience after experience, he will be able to introject this ability to think (*alpha function*), which Bion considers one of the fundamental links between human beings and which he considers to be fundamental for the development of the mind.

Thinking means trying to know the emotional experience aroused by the encounter with the other; it implies a desire and an effort to know (K) that is rooted in very early communication between mother and infant and it indicates making links, including the link between the parents.

In this theoretical system which underlies thinking, Bion hypothesises that the infant has an inborn disposition corresponding to an expectation of a breast, a *pre-conception,* and when this pre-conception is brought into contact with a *realisation* that approximates to it, the mental outcome is a conception" (1962, p. 111). He also suggests that a *thought* is originated by a frustration, by the mating of a preconception with a frustration, with an "absent breast" or "no breast" (p. 111).

When we speak of a "breast", we refer to a "function" that is carried out by the maternal container. (Bion 1962a, 1962b). Containment has three main components: firstly receptivity, the mother must be open to the emotional communication of the infant; secondly transformation, in which course the mother's *reverie*—her particular sensitivity in receiving and interpreting the infant's needs, expressed through projective identification—acting on beta elements, the inchoate sense impressions—to generate meaning; and the third is 'publication', by which the result of the transformation is communicated.

In the process of unconscious *reverie,* fundamental for the establishment of the infant's emotional development, the mother's bond with the child's father, the presence of the third and the father in the mother's mind, takes a central role.

In this respect, Meltzer describes the need for maternal and paternal functions which produce the experience of a "combined object" in the development of the child. The bisexual characteristic of the object is, according to Meltzer, that of the breast and the nipple, which are both receptive and penetrating, cosy and limiting. The lack of these characteristics gives rise to confusion over the nature of objects (Meltzer 1967, 1973).

Recognition of the bond shared by the parents outlines a limiting boundary which creates what Britton describes as a "triangular space", "a space bounded by three persons of the oedipal situation and all their potential relationships" (Britton, 1989, p. 86). As a consequence of a failure of maternal containment, according to Britton a defensive phantasy is created within the child, that he refers to as 'Oedipal illusions' which oppose the psychic reality of the oedipal situation, as well as the recognition of the nature of the relationship between the parents and therefore of the rivalry with one of them for possession of the other.

Klein had spoken of excessive projective identification, which confuses the distinction between the self and the external object (Klein, 1946; Bion, 1962b) and consequently obstructs the perception of *two-ness*, since such an awareness depends on the recognition of a distinction between subject and object.

Meltzer suggests calling this omnipotent phantasy 'intrusive identification', to highlight the invasive element and to distinguish it from the form of projective identification described by Bion, which instead is necessary for development and is a useful means of communication between mother and child.

Meltzer also explores what occurs within the object that is invaded and describes the ways in which the maternal container becomes a *claustrum*: the representation of the internal space of the mother's body, subdivided into various compartments, in which the child satisfies the need to intrude and be confused (Meltzer, 1986, 1992).

In a very interesting work, a contemporary analyst and friend of Bion and Meltzer, Roger Money-Kyrle (1968) takes up Bion's theory on the development of thought and shares his notion of an innate preconception mating with a realisation to form a conception, but uses it to show his perspective on the theory of cognitive development.

Alongside the development of a concept of a breast or of a nipple, according to Money-Kyrle, "we may suppose the development of a concept of something which receives and contains the nipple, that is a mouth…" (p. 419). Within these two innate basic preconceptions, according to the author, further differentiations take place: in the first months of life, in fact, the child learns to understand the basic structure of all those that he considers the fundamental *"facts of life"*: that is, the relationship between his parents which implies genital gratification, the fact that he was born from this relationship and is dependent on them and that other babies, his rivals, were born of it.

In his evocative description, Money-Kyrle imagines the development of a base, from breast or nipple to mother as a whole person, to the combined parents and the idea of home and a country one belongs to and so on "but environmental deficiency on the one hand, or some innate factor such as excessive envy or intolerance to frustration on the other, may interfere with the conceptual process and lead to the formation of *misconceptions*" (1965b, p. 395).

Rather than referring to the psychotic mechanisms that attack this "concept building" and make it impossible to think, as they were described by Bion, Money-Kyrle reflects on those less severe disorders which distort concepts rather than prevent their formation, and which especially distort them in order to evade the Oedipus Complex.

His interest lies in understanding the reasons for the failure that leads the child, as well as the patient in the course of analytic work, not to *recognise* what is too painful and he thinks that when a concept is not available to complete an act of *recognition*, its place is usually taken by a *misconception*.

Like Bion and Meltzer, Money-Kyrle too believes that the human being is born with a predisposition to know the truth, meaning the truth about himself, and that the impediments to its realisation are mainly emotional. From this assumption he attempts to show his theory about the oscillation between our perception of truth and the desire to distort it, taking into account those 'unconscious (non-psychotic) delusions', in particular *"disorientation and misconceptions"* (1968, pp. 417–423).

I will attempt to show, through the clinical material of the analysis of these two young children, how their thinking processes became distorted, giving rise to misconceptions which led to a breakdown in their emotional and cognitive development. Their understanding of the nature of the world is distorted by a specific failure in containment based on intrusive maternal identifications with which the child identifies. I would also attempt to illustrate how, through analysis, these children begin to rediscover the *concept*, and the initial base from which all others derive.

First clinical example

Andrew, aged five, communicated his suffering with every part of his body. He was one of those young patients whose pain would linger within me for a long time after the end of our sessions. His eyes, framed by deep dark circles, revealed sleepless nights and were able to rest on mine only after a long time, and only then was I able to see their intense blue colour. His thin body was in constant motion, I would say "on the run": Andrew felt surrounded by enemies and argued with them day and night.

In the initial phase of analysis—four sessions per week—Andrew would always rush into the room before me, and when I entered I would find him seated at the table, engrossed in making two animals fight violently, generally the dinosaur against the tiger.

He does not look at me and does not respond either to my greetings or to my short comments, which limit themselves to describing this fight, and feelings of anger and confusion. The fight continues for a long time during sessions, and Andrew emits only sounds of kicks or punches. He is pale and his face communicates an unspeakable suffering. I feel as if for Andrew I am not there.

During sessions, he would suddenly stand up and hide his face in his hands, turning to the window with his back to me. In a very aggressive tone, but whispering, he would say things like: "John fuck you!"…"Boobs, boobs…you know what boobs are… Charlotte hasn't got a boyfriend … she's a good friend…She's very pretty, she's blonde…she's got blue eyes…She's got two small, black dots … ". Andrew's expression is tense, fearful and anguished.

I look for ways to enter his desperation and to find words to describe his early anxieties which to me seem to be imbued with an exciting quality of adult sexual life. I would tell him that maybe Andrew likes Charlotte, she is blonde with blue eyes just like him, and that he also likes mummy's breast, all children like mummy's breast, it is full of good milk, but maybe Andrew feels sad because he has lost it. He suddenly takes a sheet of paper and a black marker, and with very rapid movements he draws a scribble and two black dots while saying to himself: "they are in his heart". Then he scribbles all over the drawing in black so heavily that it is completely covered up.

Then he leaves everything and once again goes to the window with his back to me, and I can understand a few words—"Leo! You mustn't call her Pupa! (which he repeats several times with an aggressive tone), You mustn't do it! Or else you know what I'll do to you! Don't you? I'll kill you! I'll get you and kill you! They'll shoot her in the boobs…they'll shoot the boobs! Leo, you are my second friend…I am a general! I'll send you to another army and I don't want to see you again!"

Andrew keeps whispering to himself walking around the room while I would comment, with a calm and concerned tone, that he is telling me that something very bad and violent has happened, something that hurts him very much. I talk to him about his wish to feel powerful like a general, and that I can understand that this is very important, because it wards off the feeling of being in danger…It's very painful to feel in danger and powerless, I know these feelings…

Andrew then takes the crocodile from the box and walks distractedly around the room holding the crocodile very tightly, muttering something I do not understand. Talking to myself, I comment that the crocodile is also strong and powerful as well as frightening and that feeling in danger and feeling that nobody can help you is the worst thing in the world. Suddenly Andrew says to himself: "squashed". I repeat "feeling squashed…yes, this is the right word!…It is a horrible feeling, feeling squashed…". At the end of our session he puts some glue on the tiger's and on the crocodile's feet and sticks them on the table. I tell him that now the tiger and the crocodile, with their anger and fears, will stay put, here with Emanuela, and that he is not alone…

History. Andrew's parents were very worried about their son, who started to behave bizarrely in the last few months. They went to a child psychiatrist for a consultation, who diagnosed "childhood schizophrenia" and wanted to put Andrew on anti-psychotic medication. At the same time, they were seeing a couple therapist for their conflictual relationship, who suggested they should get a second opinion and referred them to me.

According to the parents, Andrew was a very clever and "normal child", and they do not understand this sudden change. They tell me that they left for a few days during the summer and Andrew stayed with his grandparents in a very familiar place which he loves. However, the mother thinks that something must have happened during this time which traumatised him, and she hints at sexual games with older children or something that he saw, like a pornographic film, which might have shocked him. On their return, he almost stopped talking to them, does not pay attention to anything, does not want to go back to school, and he feels that he is surrounded by people who wants to kill him.

When mother tells me of her relationship with her child, I am struck by the language she uses, which to me has adult connotations: "we were a couple", "we travelled together all over the world" and "he adores my breast".

Andrew was the couple's first and deeply desired child. The mother's expression suddenly changes when she tells me that she is very independent and wanted to go back to work, and to smoke, and to drink... the paediatrician told her to wean the baby all in one go, and so after five months she did. Andrew suffered a lot and so did she; she cries as she remembers her baby screaming while being held by the nanny, and having to go on the balcony in order to not to see him crying and having to be separated from him, because if she heard him crying she would lose some of her milk, which would start flowing". This story is very painful, and it is clear that the mother did not and does not feel she is receiving any support from Andrew's father who appears a rather anxious man and at that time he had serious financial problems. However, the mother repeats several times that everything always went very well and this declaration strikes me, to the detriment of the words used, as a powerful and unapproachable communication which I connect to the "ghosts" which dwell in a family (Fraiberg, 1975). Ghosts which in my counter-transference, seem to be linked with mother's early sexual experiences, possibly to sexual harassment.

We agree to start intensive work, and to wait before giving him any medication.

After about two months of analysis, in a session, I watch the usual fight between the animals but at a certain point, Andrew suddenly produces a different sound, no longer of a clash but something that sounds like "perel chan chun perelenpertrlr...", and that he repeats to himself. Sitting in front of him on the small chair, I try to imitate the sound. Andrew stops and for the first time he looks at me for a second. I tell him it is a nice sound...the tongue goes up and down...it is pleasant. I repeat it. Andrew then resumes the fight between the tiger and the dinosaur but less violently, and makes another louder sound, marking the time: "dumba dum...". I observe that it sounds like a drum as I repeat it, and I say that perhaps he feels as if there is a war, and that it must be very frightening.

The dinosaur attacks the tiger, grabs it by the neck and then bites into it with its mouth, to strangle it with its curled tail. In the meantime Andrew has gotten up and continues to make the animals fight as if they were chasing each other on the walls of the room. At one point it seems that the tiger has disappeared and Andrew says "Abracadabra". The tiger reappears and the fight resumes, but the dinosaur is hit and falls to the ground. I comment on what I have observed and I ask what happened to the dinosaur. Andrew says "he lost the fight". I ask if Andrew feels sorry about this. He stands up and as if he were talking to himself, while facing the wall, he says he likes the gorilla. I tell him that the gorilla has remained in its box.

From the technical point of view, it seems impossible to pull him out of this persecutory world. His body tension conveys the feeling of someone who feels trapped and hopeless and tries to resist. I take his fantasies at face value and I say, for instance, that "since Leo and Charlotte have made him very angry, they must have done something really bad, and that I am interested in knowing what they have done…really terrible and violent things could happen and Andrew is afraid of them". Or "This Leo is really silly, and who knows why Leo and Charlotte do these things which really annoy Andrew and hurt him so much… and then he has frightening thoughts and feels like he is in danger". At times it seems to me that my words reach him, and that the intensity of his rage diminishes.

Around the third month of analysis, some changes take place. In one session, he takes from the box a brown plasticine ball made of all the colours mixed together, which he also had used to smear the walls of the room. Now he rolls it out but then leaves it. He then takes an orange-coloured piece of play-dough and divides it in half to make what look like two sticks, and puts them side-by-side. I watch him and tell him that today he does not want to make the room dirty … now there are two, they are the same and I comment on what a lovely colour he has chosen. I add that they look very pretty and probably feel happy to be so close!…They are close but not confused. Like a child next to his mother…like Andrew and Emanuela here. Andrew leaves the session calm and smiling.

Gradually Andrew appears more in touch with reality most of the time; he is able to stay in class and in the sessions he likes engaging with me and he is now able to look at me. Mother decides to begin individual therapy.

On one occasion, while lying on the bed, playing with his chewing gum, Andrew puts it under his upper lip, looks at me and says "I've got braces". We both laugh. He becomes curious and looks around as he walks calmly into the room; or on his way to the toilet, he tries to open the other doors and asks me what is there, and how many children I have. At times he looks calmly at old pictures he drew and comments on them. He also starts to draw some simple human figures and then also some large round faces, some with visible teeth. I comment on his being interested in his mouth, which contains braces and teeth which can bite, but at the same time they can hold on to something important without letting it go. Andrew takes the gorilla and starts jumping around the room making noises such as "Uuh Uuh!... Me Gorilla!" walking towards me. I tell him that the gorilla was in the box, but now he comes towards me, and perhaps wishes to tell me something that I am very interested to hear. Using the play-dough he makes what he calls a big brown sausage, which he then transforms into a gun, says "fire" and then other swear words. I tell him that this large scary gorilla is perhaps hungry, and would like a large sausage for his large teeth. On another occasion, he puts two rubber balls underneath his shirts and laughs, saying "the king of bubs!".

In the next session, he takes the shark, which also has large teeth, and makes it swim in the blue basin where there is some water. He then lies on the bed and pretends to swim too for a few moments. He swims in a calm way and seems to enjoy it. I comment that there is a place here for the 'shark-feelings' of Andrew and he feels he can swim safely.

Later on in this session, he will tell me about the friends he has lost (when he changed school) and about his jealousy towards his little brother. We can now talk about the feelings he experiences on days when we do not meet, and how desperate and angry he feels when he thinks he has lost something which means so much to him.

Andrew also tells me his first bad dream in which he is falling and ending up in hospital. I talk to him about his fear of being dropped from my mind during the long weekend in which we are not going to meet. He listens, and while sitting in front of me, he takes off his shoe and tries to put something inside it. When I comment that the shoe seems to be a safe place, Andrew says "tortoise". The gorilla and now the tortoise seem the only two possibilities to deal with feeling of helplessness.

In the next weeks he starts a particular game. It seems he wants to build something. Over the course of various sessions, he devotes particular attention to putting the small table and the two small chairs in different positions; it seems he has an idea in mind. After having turned the table upside down, he finally manages to create a living space between the four upturned table-legs, with a couple of cushions and the blanket. He looks at me for a while, explaining to me how the boat works and how to get into it. I am very curious and ask him for details. Andrew mimes rowing with one oar to one side, then with two oars and then he explains that there can be a boat wheel and that I can use an engine. He is very sweet. He then tells me that at some point a big wave could arrive, and then a shark too...I therefore ask him what he would do then, what to do if he is in danger. Andrew says that there is a sat-nav that tells you if the sea is rough and after a pause he then adds: "Call father... Daddy come here...". Then he wants to put the blanket over the top to make a tent and asks me to help him. I help him and then tell him it looks really nice and that it feels like a very safe place, and this is also because he feels daddy protects him, and that he is not alone. Andrew goes inside the boat and looks out, smiling and satisfied.

A container takes shape, a new conception of a container, a boat and a father who can protect him. In this period, the father reports that Andrew had whispered something in his ear: he had said that he did not want anybody to hear what he had to tell him and so the father decided to hide with Andrew in a small storeroom with the light on, and told Andrew that he could talk there as nobody would hear them. Andrew then said: "let's hide the dummy". So they put it in the strong box to keep it safe.

After about a year, Andrew's behaviour is back to normal. He happily goes to school and tells me about the things that happen to him and about the emotions he feels.

In one session, he begins to play a new game: It starts off like "hide and seek"; I have to look around the room for him, after having counted while sitting on my chair with my eyes closed. He generally hides under the bed or behind the curtain. I slowly wander around the room and search for him. He is happy to be found, and hardly ever asks me to hide.

At a certain point, along the course of our sessions, after playing the usual hide-and-seek for a while, he hides behind my chair, crouching low, and I have to find him by moving my arms behind me. I pretend to be surprised and a bit like in the Hansel and Gretel story, and when he puts a pen in my hand, I say, "No, it's not Andrew! It's too hard and small". Then I move my hands again, trying to touch his face, and he places a little car in my hand. After a few tries he lets my hand touch his forehead and enthusiastically, I state that I have found somebody! I touch him gently (he is always behind me, silent and calm) and slowly, with my finger, I then touch his nose and move down to his lips, which I trace very delicately. For several sessions I try to think about the meaning of this game which, to me, seems to convey feelings of very early experiences. At some point, one day, as I touch his lips he says: "It's me!" and wants me to continue and to repeat the game many times and for a long time. Each time I touch his lips, Andrew repeats: "This is me!".

I thought that Andrew was communicating something about feeling *recognised* and the possibility of having his own identity and to be unique.

Discussion: Initially, I thought that Andrew found himself inside a *claustrum* (Meltzer, 1992), where he moved from being 'the king of bubs' in the upper compartment, to being trapped in an anal world where everything is ruined, feeling like the unclean faecal ball with which he dirtied the walls of the room, and with an enormous rage inside.

The breakdown occurred on a weekend when Andrew probably found himself involved in a world of sexuality with older children, in the absence of his parents, but that particular situation reactivated the old trauma of a weaning where the breast/mother disappears, overwhelming him with anger at this sexualised mother who betrays him.

Initially Andrew faces his feeling of helplessness, of feeling 'squashed', with his childish omnipotence, which makes him feel that he is the general with the qualities of a crocodile, and this makes him feel safe. (Symington, 1985).

The *misconception* leads the child to have a belief: that he is the mother's partner and that babies should excite mothers. This distorted picture seems to have been initiated by the mother who, through intrusive identification, conveys to the child her confusion, and is unable to help him to gradually absorb the reality of the oedipal configuration. The difficulties encountered in this relationship are significantly increased by the absence of the paternal figure, both in reality and in the mind of the mother.

However, Andrew manages to move on from there: he discovers the idea that it is possible to be two, together but not confused, that this is a way in which he can feel better. The good-nourishing breast is now rediscovered as the way for new preconceptions to encounter adequate conceptions.

Second clinical example[1]

Edward, aged four, in analysis for three sessions per week.

Edward's parents were referred by the child neuropsychiatric service, whom they had approached, owing to language difficulties when the child was three years old. In the first months of school, the teachers were alarmed because the child did not speak, was not able to be with others, and tended to isolate himself or run around in circles in the room. He showed muscle stiffness, and on the basis of these signs, a diagnosis of autism spectrum disorder was hypothesised. The child underwent speech therapy, but the sounds were still metallic and echolalic, difficult to understand. After a year, following the suggestion of another child psychiatrist, the parents decided to consult another neuropsychiatrist, who advised them to begin a course of psychoanalytic psychotherapy.

History. Edward was breastfed for around 15 months, before going straight to drinking from a glass. At the time of weaning, his mother lost her mother who had seriously ill for several months and that since mother was leaving in another country, she could not assist her.

The meeting with the parents revealed a development that was neither very gradual, nor particularly modulated. It is the father, who during the meeting was able to emphasise the fact that mother and son had spent much time together, in a relationship which left little room for anything, or anyone else. He shared, with regret, the fact that, owing to work, he travels a lot and is present at home only on weekends and even then not always.

For the first three months of analysis, Edward wanted his mother to enter the room with him, and to sit in her lap. After three months, he began to play with the therapist, but only in the presence of the mother. He gradually agreed to the mother sitting in the waiting room, but she had to accompany him into the room and then take him at the end of the session. His favourite game was to tie every object in the room with sticky tape and create a kind of cobweb which also make it difficult to move. He gradually began to play and build a garage or house, within which he made a small blue car go up and down.

After about eight months of analysis, he began to be more curious about the consulting room and looked around rather than racing in as usual; he began to speak about his grandmother, the mother of the father who he was very fond of, and of the father who sometimes told him "no" when he could not do things.

In one session, for the first time Edward built two objects that could move - a train and a submarine. The analyst noted that they can explore the marine world and the world above water, and that the train can also transport many things and people. In this session, for the first time he did not want the mother to enter the room and take him. He got dressed by himself, and once he was ready to leave, he approached his mother, took her hand and brought his head close to her arm, and while looking at her, he said: "I like you". The mother looked at him, smiling, and told him: "I like you too".

After about a year of analysis, for the first time the analyst had to skip the previous session and Monday was a holiday, so they met again on Thursday after a week.

The analyst told Edward, "Today we meet again after not meeting for a few days, we missed each other but together we rediscovered your games and you continued with your beautiful constructions".

The boy nodded and shortly afterwards told her that today he would like to "fix the cars".

He took the big truck, the one we often called 'mummy truck' in the past, which he had not played with for a while. He took it and fixed it with some tools. He also hammered it a few times a little harder.

The analyst commented that he had not played with the truck for a long time, that today he wanted to fix it but also gave it a few stronger blows, perhaps because Edward was a little angry today.

The child continued with his repairs for a little longer, then picked up a white lorry that he had coloured completely with pink marker at some point earlier and told her, "I would like to clean the truck, let's go to the bathroom and wash it…I want it to be like it was before". They went to the bathroom and the boy washed the truck with great care. He covered it with soap several times, washed it thoroughly and carefully, and said to it, "Now I'll wash the wheels, now I'll wash the top". Then he dried the truck carefully. The analyst's impression as she saw Edward taking care of the truck was similar to seeing a nurse washing a newborn baby. It was a very intense and delicate moment.

As they walked back to the room, the boy stopped for a moment in the corridor and showing the analyst the truck said: "It looks like a double-decker bus… I once saw one with my dad and he told me that one day he would take me for a ride". The analyst told him that the double-decker bus made her think of a space that gets bigger, from one to two floors and can hold many people.

At the end of the session Edward put the little blue car on the table and said that he wanted it to stay there.

In the next session Edward said that he would like to make a slide out of sticky tape. He asked for help to make it. The slide went from the back of the chair, which was higher, to the table below. First the child made the analyst place a strip of sticky tape. He fetched the blue car and tried to make it slide. It did not work because only one strip of tape was too weak to hold the car, and it was not thick enough to hold both wheels. He realised that he needed to add more strips. After several attempts and the addition of several strips of scotch tape, the slide held. Edward was jubilant when the car slid down without falling for the first time.

He told the analyst that he would like to leave the slide and find it again next session. She told him that it was not possible, as he knew well, but that perhaps he was asking her if together they could find a way to keep this slide which was so precious to him. She said that perhaps they could work out together how to keep it even if we did not leave it in that position. She said that maybe the slide could be taped and removed. The boy, after protesting at first, listened to her and commented. "Yes, it can be taken off and put back, we won't throw it away". "We wouldn't throw it away", she said.

After this exchange, Edward went to collect the constructions made during the previous sessions. He placed them on the carpet. They were a garage, a submarine and a train. The boy admired them for a while, said something that sounded like "I am", which conveyed a power which was different from the omnipotence shown in the past, as if the objects he had made said something about him. For a while he looked at the small container in the garage, checking that the pieces he had put inside were still there. Everything seemed to have held up quite well.

He then announced that he was very thirsty. He carefully poured some water into the glass and, unlike other times, stopped. It seemed that this sip of water would be enough, and that he did not need to drink the entire contents of the glass, or drink and drink again as the analyst saw him do voraciously in the past. He stopped and told that he would drink the remaining water next time. He looked at the therapist, who smiled at him.

He then said he wanted to repair the cars. He actually picked up the blue car, looked at it closely and noticed that there was a number printed on the bonnet: "911". He said that he would like to write 911 on the roof of the car and on the side as well. He took a piece of paper, asked the analyst to write 911 and to stick it on the car. The analyst commented that Edward wanted to give a sort of identity to the car, as if from now on the car would stop being an ordinary car and become a 911 car.

During the following session Edward, once alone, asked the analyst, "How come we didn't meet on Tuesday?". She commented that he was thinking about Tuesday's session, that he had thought about it a lot during the previous sessions as well, and that he wanted to know why it had not been possible to meet. She added that maybe he did not know whether she was in the room or not and perhaps he feared that she had met other children while she was not with him. He nodded. She told him that when she could not meet him there was no one in his place, that when they had sessions (she specified our days and times) no one could take his place. She explained to him that the Tuesday they skipped, she did not work, that she was not in her office.

After her comment he said, "You were not in the room". She told him that he was right, that on Tuesday we did not meet, and that she was not in the room. He continued telling her, "You didn't play with another child and nobody could touch my box …. and I can't touch another child's box". She told him that it was exactly like that and that today he thought he could ask me these things, that he knew she was interested in his questions and that she could understand that some things were difficult for him.

He then went to his little box and took out the sticky tape slide that he had made with her during the previous sessions. This time he attached the slide but did not make any cars slide on it. He left the slide in that position and went back to his box. He took the water bottle, poured the water into the glass up to the brim without letting a single drop of water out of the glass. He was very careful and then announced to her, "OK I was very thirsty, but now it's OK and I'll drink this water next week". He fetched two more cars from the box and wanted that the analyst write the numbers on pieces of paper, even though he could write the various numbers, as if somehow, this is what the analyst found herself thinking, that this 'christening' had to involve an adult.

The analyst told him that he was trying to tell her that he too wanted to be as unique as the cars, that he too wanted to be just him rather than being another child.

Edward remained on the carpet a little longer and moved his cars. He looked at them for a long time and seemed pleased. Suddenly he got up and came towards her, stood next to her table and with considerable uncertainty asked her this question, "But did mummy eat me to put me in her tummy? But when did she eat me? When I was one or two years old?"

She told him that mothers do not eat babies, that no mother eats her own baby and that is not the way babies end up in the tummy. He said, "Mothers don't eat babies?". Again she told him that mothers do not eat babies, and she mentioned fathers, to explain to him that it is fathers and mothers together who put them in the tummy and that babies do not enter through the mouth.

He commented, "But it's like a little door that stays open?". The analyst told him that it is like a little door that opens to make room for a baby but she also pointed out that it closes again, and that the mother's belly does not stay open.

He then said, "But then I wasn't one or two years old!". The analyst told him no, that he was not one or two years old, that he was really microscopic in his mother's tummy and that he stayed there for nine months to grow, and that when he was ready, his mother gave birth to him. He said, "But then I was zero years old?". The analyst said yes, he was zero years old. The time was over, they put the toys away and headed for his mother. When Edward reunited with his mother, he hugged her and said, "Thank you for not eating me!".

Discussion

Edward's thinking process is distorted by his phantasy that not sticking to the object, means to be aborted and thrown away. As with Andrew, the mother plays a central role in it; she finds difficult being separate from the child and forming a couple with the father.

Edward does not know when he was born, when he was 'eaten', whether it was at one or two years of age. This is the period of his weaning and it is as if his trying to clear up this confusion, as if he would say: "But did mummy eat me when she was supposed to let me go?!". Edward's mother was unable to mourn her own mother, and upon having breastfed him for 15 months, was unable to help him explore the world.

When he carefully created a slide with the tape, he shows his discovery that the link with the loved object can be maintained without being stuck to it. This is a time when the presence of the father arrives with the double-decker bus. Edward now can wait to find his mother and analyst again, and he can also wait to finish drinking the water another time— there will be time. He can talk because a sense of time and space develops when Edward is no longer sticky, which was his way of facing the feeling of helplessness.

Thinking about the diagnosis of autistic spectrum disorder and the failure to develop language, Edward seems to re-discover in his analysis the child before 15 months, the beginning of his life.

Like Andrew, at the end of a year of psychoanalysis, Edward begins to be curious and inquisitive, to look around rather than hurrying into the room, to observe and ask questions. Both patients seem to be wondering after the first year: what is reality? Reality is no longer taken for granted and they are open to curiosity and desire for knowledge (K). They discover, or re-discover, the object, not a *misconception*.

The old theory about the world is disrupted and a new reality is established. The boat and the double-decker bus are the expression of a new space, a triangular space, and of a new object to discover, that will inevitably lead to new turbulence during the course of the analysis.

Conclusion

The psychoanalytic work with Andrew and Edward seemed to me to reveal an intrinsic function in their developmental breakdown, that is, to express the need to go back in order to go forward. Being able to go back meant tracing the nature of the *misconceptions* generated by an intrusive maternal identification and recovering their true meaning.

These two young patients were referred to analysis at five and four years old, respectively, with two frightening diagnoses: infantile schizophrenia and autistic spectrum disorder. At a certain point in their childhood it was no longer possible to move forward, to deal with the separation from their mother, to relate to their peers, to be open to learning and to explore the world.

In relation to the fear of breakdown during analysis, Winnicott (1974) thinks that the patient has not actually experienced the trauma because the ego at that time was underdeveloped and unstable, and therefore he needs to experience the trauma in the transference with the analyst for the first time. I partially agree with this perspective, as I feel the original trauma has been fully experienced by the infant or children, although the memories are located in their body.

It also seems to me that the failure in maternal containment I describe, could not be thought of as the "reverse of the container/contained" relationship described by Williams (1997) and referring to a "child used as a receptacle for maternal projective identifications". The author uses "No-Entry" to describe these types of defences, which are frequently seen in patients with eating disorders and which are developed in an attempt to metabolise the unprocessed maternal projections.

The young patients I describe, and the others I have in mind, initially appear to be somewhat seduced by the maternal projections that distort the *"facts of life"*. These altered facts are that "you and I will be together for ever and ever and there is no other"; therefore the child's preconception of a containing breast is somehow relinquished and transformed in: "I don't need to be dependent on an object as we are all one". Either he possesses and intrusively identifies with the object, or he is intruded and swallowed by it. There is no sense of time and space, no frustrations that inevitably exist in any container-contained relationship.

This wrong theory about existence, this shared illusion of an absence of a 'triangular space' is disrupted at the time in which the encounter with reality inevitably clashes with this distorted image of the world. The child's pseudo-adaptability to the environment—so that many parents describe as "normal" their children's development—could be the reason for problems arising only at puberty, when the reality of bodily changes overturns the idea of control and possession (Laufer, 1986). In my clinical experience, I have often noticed that it is this distortion of thought processes that forms the basis of developmental breakdown during adolescence and which are grounded in an altered development of primary processes such as faulty splitting and projective/introjective mechanisms which lead to intrusive identifications rather than to projective identification, necessary for primary communication and for emotional and mental development.

The unbearable feelings of loss which Andrew and Edward experienced around weaning (Klein, 1936) at five and 15 months, respectively, was even more traumatic as a result of *misconceptions and disorientations* regarding the maternal containment function. The role the child plays in the mother's phantasy, interferes with the space he needs to discover and he ends up identifying with the intruder because this is the only way of relating that he knows. Such 'identification with the intruder' allows him to survive *nothingness*, the maternal impossibility of *reverie* mainly, owing to the absence of a loving presence from the father both in reality and in the mother's mind.

The notions of container (Bion, 1962a and 1962b), as well as that of psychic skin (Bick, 1968) or psychic envelope (Anzieu, 1995) imply a psychic bisexuality (Meltzer, 1973) of the primitive levels of identifications with qualities of receptivity and flexibility, together with the paternal function of solidity and setting limits. A gradual improvement has also occurred in both children's analysis, owing to the therapy undergone by both mothers and parental couples.

This theoretical framework appears useful to me for thinking in terms of what disturbs the developmental processes, and seeing *breakdown* in a new light, as it involves a broader consideration of the misunderstandings which can severely distort the structure of cognitive development. I very much agree with Meltzer, in that I find "the particular charm" of this concept (1981) to lie in its non-judgemental quality.

In the meeting with the analyst there is a discovery of a new relationship and a new perspective of the world, by means of the development of a sense of time and space for imagination (Winnicott, 1953), as well as allowing the child's freedom to get to know the object and develop a capacity to use it (Winnicott, 1968).

During the first year of analysis, it was possible for these young patients to re-discover the development of a *base*, from the breast/nipple towards the mother as a whole person, and towards the parents as a "combined object". There are new identifications, as well as a new space for thinking (Money-Kyrle, 1968).

By means of an analytical relationship, the passage from a *breakdown* to a *breakthrough* (Bion, 1965) occurs through the recognition of a new interpretation of reality, which creates the basis for the development of a sense of identity.

Note

1 I am most grateful to Dr Angela Salina, whose work I supervise, for having granted me permission to present the clinical material of her young patient.

References

Alhanati, S. 2002. *Primitive Mental States*, Karnac.

Alvarez, A. 1992. *'A developmental view of 'defence' in Live Company*, Routledge.

Anzieu, D. 1995. *Le Moi-peau*. Paris, Dunod.

Bick, E. 1968. The experience of the skin in early object relations. *Int. J. Psychoanal.* 49: 484–486.

Bion, W. 1962a. *Learning from experience*, London, Heinemann.

Bion, W. 1962b. *'A theory of thinking' in Second Thoughts*, London, Heinemann.

Bion, W. 1965. *Transformations*, London, Karnac.

Britton, R. 1989. The missing link: parental sexuality in the Oedipus Complex. In *The Oedipus Complex Today. Clinical implications.* Karnac Books.

Fraiberg, S. 1975. Ghosts in the nursery: a psychoanalytic approach to the problems of impaired infant-mother relationships, *J. Of the American Academy of Child Psychiatry*, vol. 14, no. 3.

Fraiberg, S. 1982. Pathological Defences in Infancy , *The Psychoanalytic Quarterly*, 51: 612–635.

Freud, S. 1985. *The Complete Letters of Sigmund Freud to Wilhelm Fleiss, 1887–1904*.

Klein, M. 1936. *'Weaning' The Writings of Melanie Klein*, Vol 1. The Hogarth Press.

Klein, M. 1946. *Notes on some Schizoid Mechanisms*, Vol 1. The Hogarth Press.

Klein, M. 1959. *'Our adult world and its roots in infancy' The writings of Melanie Klein*, Vol. III, The Hogarth Press.

Laufer, M. and Laufer, E. 1986. *Adolescenza e breakdown evolutivo*, Bollati Boringhieri.

Mancia, M. 1981. On the Beginning of Mental Life in the Foetus, *Int.l J. of Psycho-Analysis*, 62: 351–357.

Meltzer, D. 1967. *The Psychoanalytical Process*. Heinemann.

Meltzer, D. 1973. *Sexual States of Mind*, Perthshire, Clunie Press.

Meltzer, D. 1981. *'Does Money-Kyrle's concept of misconception have any unique descriptive power?' Sincerity and other works: Collected Papers of Donald Meltzer*, Karnac Books.

Meltzer, D. 1986. *Studies in Extended Metapsychology: clinical applications of Bion's ideas*, Perthshire, Clunie Press.

Meltzer, D. 1992. *The Claustrum: an investigation of claustrophobic phenomena*, Perthshire, Clunie Press.

Money-Kyrle, D. 1965. *'Success and Failure in mental maturation' Collected papers of Roger Money-Kyrle*, Clunie Press.

Money-Kyrle, R. 1965. *'Review of Bion Elements of Psychoanalysis' Collected papers of Roger Money Kyrle*. Clunie Press.

Money-Kyrle, R. 1968. *'Cognitive Developments' Collected papers of Roger Money-Kyrle*.

O'Shaughnessy, E. 2015. A Commemorative Essay on W.R. Bion's Theory of Thinking, In: *Inquiries in Psychoanalysis*, Routledge.

Quagliata, E. 2014. All'origine del dialogo tra genitori e figli. In: *Dialoghi con i genitori*, Astrolabio.

Quagliata, E. 2018. *Il breakdown evolutivo in adolescenza: conversazione con Egle Laufer*. In: *Adolescenti in crisi*, Astrolabio.

Salomonsson, B. 2016. Infantile Defences in parent-infant psychotherapy: the example of gaze avoidance, *Int. J. Psychoanal.*, 97: 65–88.

Symington, J. 1985. The Survival Function of Primitive Omnipotence, *Int. J. Psychoanal*, 66: 481–487.

Stern, D. 1985. *The Interpersonal world of the Infant*, Basic Books.

Trevarthen, C. 1979. Communication and cooperation in early infancy: a description of primary subjectivity. In: *Before speech: the beginning of interpersonal communication*. Cambridge University Press.

Tustin, F. 1988. The black hole a significant element in autism, *Free Associations*, 11: 35–50.

Williams, G. 1997. Reflections on some dynamics of eating disorders: 'no entry' defences and foreign bodies, *Int. J. Psychoanal*. 78: 927–941.

Winnicott, D. 1953. Transitional objects and transitional phenomena –a study of the first not-me possession, *Int. J. Psychoanalysis*, 34: 89–97.

Winnicott, D. 1968. The use of an object and relating through identification, *Int. J. Psychoanalysis*, 50[1969]: 711.

Winnicott, D. 1974. Fear of Breakdown , *Int. Review of Psychoanal.*, 1: 103–107.

10 Repairing a Fractured Child and Family Mind

Caroline Sehon

Introduction

What are the explicit and implicit theories that inform ways of under-standing and working analytically with couples and families? What ratio-nales do we rely on to recommend one specific therapy or combination of therapies over another? This paper illustrates how link and field theories lend a way of listening and integrating clinical data from parallel child and couple therapy tracks.

Link and field theories are explicated in *The Interpersonal Unconscious* (Scharff and Scharff, 2011). From an object relations perspective, each family member's voice speaks primarily for that person's unconscious. Traditionally, this theoretical dimension has underemphasised the uncon-scious organisation residing within the social links *between* marital part-ners and *among* family members. In contrast, *link theory*, as conceived in the 1950s by Enrique Pichon-Rivière (a Swiss-born Argentinean psycho-analyst), regards each family member as also communicating the family's interpersonal unconscious, which resides within the interactive space among family members (Pichon-Rivière, 1956/1957). This unconscious register is formed by *el vinculo* (links), which represent, for example, trau-matic material, affects, and recurrent relational patterns. Links are trans-mitted unconsciously via 1) a vertical dimension, between prior and current generations; and 2) a horizontal dimension, among current-day family members, friends, and their broader social group. Together, these links form an overarching structure within the family that shapes, and is shaped by, each family member. Additionally, these links exist within the consulting room in a space between patient and analyst, or between the couple and analyst.

In the early 1960s the Argentinean psychoanalysts Madeleine and Willy Baranger applied the concept of the *field* to the analytic situation. The Barangers were influenced by Freud, Pichon-Rivière, Kurt Lewin and Maurice Merleau-Ponty from gestalt psychology, and object relationists–particularly Melanie Klein, Susan Isaacs and Wilfred Bion (Baranger, 2005; Baranger and Baranger, 2008). The connections between concepts arising

DOI: 10.4324/9781003246749-10

from object relations, link theory, and field theory are discussed in Scharff and Scharff (2011). This theoretical lens informs an analytic approach to working with a family in multiple therapy contexts. In this way, the clinician has a greater opportunity to restructure existing links and unchain the family from their traumatic, intergenerational relational patterns. Accordingly, a synergy can be gained that might be missed with less intensive therapeutic strategies.

Characters in the field

The term "characters in the field" was coined by Ferro (2009). The main characters of this family are the children, Britney and Lionel; their parents, Gabrielle and Maddox; and the children's grandmothers and deceased grandfathers. Britney is a ten-year-old bright, creative, and dramatic child. Her parents brought her to me, seeking help for her anxiety, sadness, loneliness, moodiness, temper tantrums, and hypersexuality. Her six-year-old brother, Lionel, also had anxiety, and his hyperactivity and defiant storms often overtook the family. Britney and Lionel had formed an intense love–hate relationship, in which they were sometimes caught in the midst of a French kiss, romantic embrace, or (less commonly), heated brawl.

The parents' marital difficulties were initially obscured from my view. Gabrielle works as a real estate agent. She is forthright, articulate, and psychologically minded. She and Maddox have been married 19 years. Maddox is an athletic, short-statured man. He is employed as a surveillance officer in the army; as such, he is frequently called to emergencies and national disasters. The youngest of three, Maddox was scarred by a childhood in which he was tortured by two older cousins, harshly disciplined by his father, and unprotected by his controlling and critical mother. He left home bereft of a good internal parental couple. In his early adult years, he lost his father unexpectedly to suicide, a tragic event that haunts him and for which he blames himself. Also the youngest of three, Gabrielle described her childhood as free of trauma, though she recalls suffering with depression and anxiety as a child. She too internalised a fractured parental couple. As a young adult, she felt shattered by the sudden loss of her father and paternal grandfather, being deeply attached to both. Later she took on a parentified role in relation to her mother.

Therapeutic Approach

My work with the family over several years began with an individual psychoanalytic therapy for Britney, combined with parent guidance work. During this initial phase of our journey, Britney made steady progress, despite strain within her parents' relationship. Gradually, I saw the extent of the couple's difficulties, which they could no longer hide from me or from themselves.

Gabrielle and Maddox were often at war with each other over their dissonant parenting approaches. They felt unable to get past the aftermath of the traumatic losses of their fathers. Their intimate emotional and sex life had run aground. As I listened to the unconscious dynamics reverberating within the couple field, I became aware of parallel links that informed Britney's unconscious fantasy life and play (Figure 10.1). I pondered two questions: Would it be therapeutically advantageous to offer couple therapy to Gabrielle and Maddox while remaining Britney's therapist, or would it be preferable for the couple to see an independent therapist? Would this shift from parent guidance to couple therapy absolutely preclude my deepening the work with the couple, or rather could it leverage the family's growth to a greater extent by virtue of my being the container for both the child and the couple, providing me access to more of the family's links? By *container*, I refer to Wilfred Bion's concept of the analyst's maternal attitude and "reverie" (Bion, 1962).

On careful reflection, I decided to offer a trial of couple therapy, whilst continuing as Britney's therapist, so long as I could hold in mind these parallel fields and maintain a clear boundary around each therapy, and provided I saw evidence that the family links were healing. The couple felt that they had secured a solid foundation of trust in me, and they opted for a trial of couple therapy with me. Several months later, the couple sought therapy for their son, Lionel, from a colleague of mine, recognising that if I had offered individual therapy to Lionel, it would have compromised the boundaries of Britney's therapy.

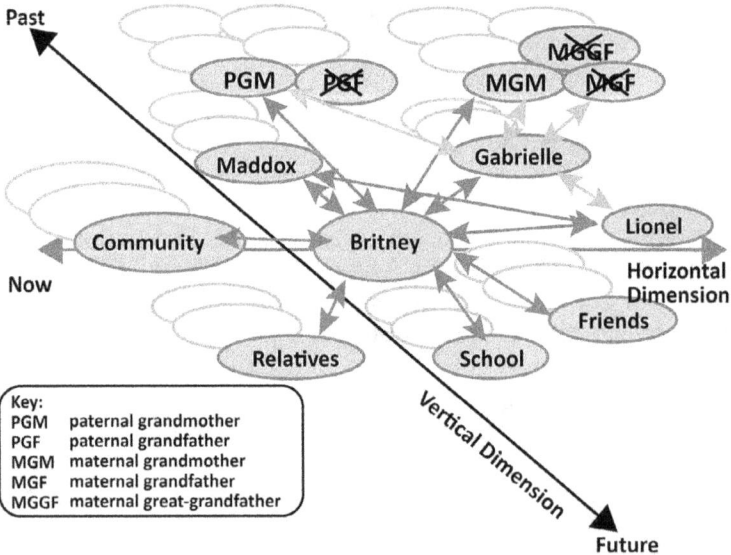

Figure 10.1 Link theory and the interpersonal unconscious
MGM=maternal grandmother; MGF=maternal grandfather; MGGF=maternal great-grandfather; PGM=paternal grandmother; PGF=paternal grandfather

Listening to links within the field

An entrée into the family's field can be seen by looking at a photograph of a Lego house created by Britney (Figure 10.2). This image is a representative example of other houses that she has drawn or built. According to link theory, this image might represent the interior of the "family mind"— that superordinate structure that Pichon-Rivière described as containing the family's multigenerational links. A relatively open interior floor plan with the barest of boundaries demarcates each room. Britney has planted a tree on the inside of (rather than outside) the house. The front door is not held securely in place by any walls or other supporting structures. This boundary confusion could be a link. The absence in Britney's house of boundaries between internal and external environments, between these separate interior spaces, illustrates the interpenetration of family members' minds. Accordingly, each family member has had difficulty developing her or his separate identity. This house also illustrates the exposure and vulnerability of its inhabitants to "ghosts" from the past that could trespass into the house and move among the minds of those dwelling in the

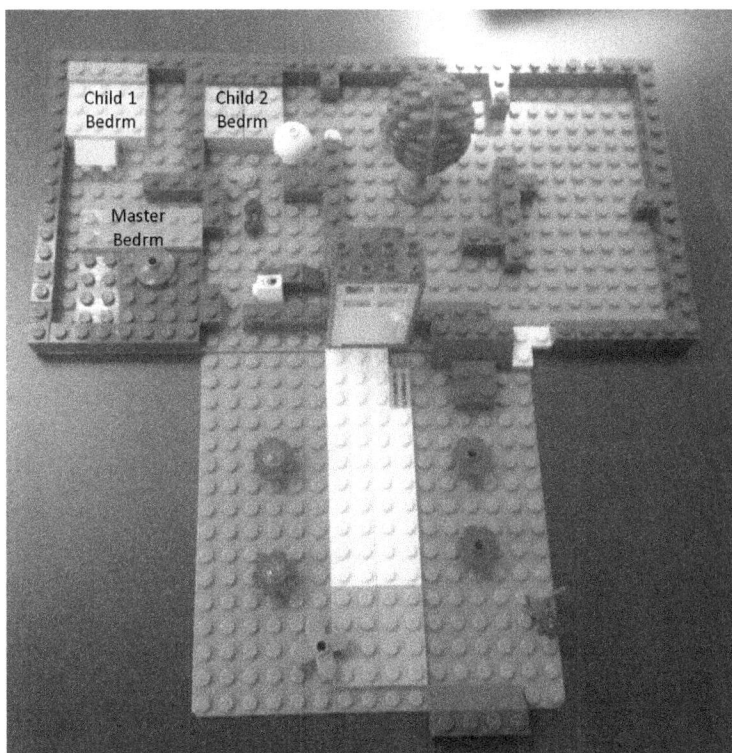

Figure 10.2 Britney's first Lego house

here-and-now. Britney and Lionel have been subject to the projections of their parents' links, namely their anxieties, fears, sexual longings, and aggressive feelings. In this family, the unconscious transmission of links has been happening for a long time without sufficient containment. Although Britney built this house on her own, out of Lego blocks, it is (according to link theory) as if the family constructed the house together, being that its creation rests on the foundation of the family's interpersonal unconscious.

In a similar vein, a dream produced by one family member carries links that could equally have been communicated unconsciously by another member, whether through a dream or some other unconscious expression. Britney dreamed:

> I just kept seeing these huge tarantulas. They were everywhere. No matter where I went, they were there. They were on my back, on the window–everywhere. Then, when I woke up, my Dad was sleeping on the couch and my brother was sleeping, so I went upstairs to sleep with my Mom. After a while, when I closed my eyes, I kept seeing the outline of a tarantula, so I kept opening my eyes.

According to object relations theory, these alien and threatening creatures could symbolise persecutory internal objects that felt invasive to Britney—"they were everywhere." This dream captures links of aggressive affects, carried by the intrusive tarantulas that force their way across time and space, barging across the barriers of generations and among the minds within her own family. At the same time, these tarantulas appear to symbolise toxic, unmetabolised, emotional material that cannot be contained by any family member and that leave each person frozen in terror, frightened that tomorrow will bring only more tragedy.

Two vignettes from the parallel tracks of couple and child therapy, at different phases of this work, exemplify the therapeutic movement that came about by listening to and interpreting the interpersonal unconscious within these two fields. At the outset of couple therapy, we worked on uncovering Gabrielle and Maddox's initial unconscious attraction to one another based on their underlying projective identificatory systems. Each partner desperately hoped to use the other to re-find their idealised fathers, whom they had lost. They projected their internal mothers onto each other. Gabrielle misidentified Maddox as being like her weak, passive, dependent mother, which led Gabrielle to become angry with him for his inadequate co-parenting. Maddox felt criticised, bullied, and controlled by Gabrielle, onto whom he projected his domineering mother and torturing cousins. He managed these transferences to her by using various distancing manoeuvres, like passively avoiding his parenting responsibilities, drug use, and exploding with aggression, which only led his wife to pull further.

During the initial phase of the couple therapy, Gabrielle and Maddox formed sibling transferences to me in which each looked to me for approval.

At these moments, I experienced them as quarrelling children. I came to recognise that my role, at times, was to serve as a new object, a differentiating third, who could help each of them to try standing alone as individuals in their own right. As to countertransference, I felt on guard, fearful that Gabrielle and Maddox could feel excluded by the other, being that they seemed to compete with each other for an exclusive partnership with me.

Initially, Gabrielle would flood the session with words, in contrast with Maddox, who communicated nonverbally. He often signalled to me that he needed to be rescued against Gabrielle's barrage of criticism, and he seemed to want me to throw him a lifeline when he did not know how to verbalise his feelings. He expressed being terrified of asserting himself, partly because he feared that this would become a slippery slope—he might become aggressive like (and more identified with) his brothers and father. I often experienced a concordant identification with Maddox, who felt crowded out by Gabrielle, and I felt pressured to make space for him to help him reclaim his voice. I learned that these heated arguments were frequent at home, but in that context, Maddox would often explode in an uncontrollable rage when he could not express himself in words.

Early in the couple work, I discovered that they had banded together (out of desperation) to hold Lionel down when he refused to take his psychiatric medication. This practice stopped when I helped them see how this incident represented a re-enactment of Maddox's childhood trauma (identification with the aggressor). This sadomasochistic pattern was echoed within the analytic field of Britney's therapy sessions. For example, she would enact similar scenarios in her play, or directly toward me (in the transference), like when she threatened me with a pair of scissors if I did not acquiesce to her demands. Hence, from my exposure to these different therapy contexts, I saw that these aggressive links were transmitted around the family like nonstop torpedoes, echoing the dramas staged within prior generations, and between past and current generations.

In the child therapy, Britney produced a one-hour video in which women competed aggressively to win a man's favours. The women passionately longed to take out the man on a date. The man ultimately fell mortally ill when he ate a meal that a feminist woman has prepared with peanuts and pollen–to which he was severely allergic, though she declares her love for him. "Poisoning" is her only way to break out of a stereotypical image of her grandmother's generation in which the woman is enslaved to the man. Interestingly, Britney creatively captures the idea of links by "poisoning" the food.

This movie can also be seen as a fractal of her general therapy. As the movie proceeded, Brittney shifted between her old, sadomasochistic model of relating to me and her more collaborative ways of working with me. For example, at first, she aggressively insisted on being scriptwriter, producer and videographer, and she crowded me out of any collaborating role. As the movie evolved, she allowed a partnership to develop, with the opening of a space within which she and I thought together about the meaning of her play.

In a parallel fashion, Gabrielle and Maddox formed a more secure partnership. Their aggression at home diminished, as Maddox learned to put his "nameless dread" into words, and Gabrielle allowed him to claim the floor for himself. As the couple's relationship stabilised, they provided their children a desperately needed container. In step, Britney's therapy deepened–she felt less sad and anxious, and more able to verbalise her distress and to reflect on her symbolic play rather than to simply enact it. She increasingly used me as a helpful object instead of assuming an independent, pseudomature position or trying to overtake me in a repetitive, sadomasochistic manner. Gradually, she developed a greater sense of herself as a unique, individual person.

Several months later, Gabrielle and Maddox were working more harmoniously as partners, both to support each other and to co-parent. For example, on one occasion, upon returning from a business trip, Maddox rushed from the airport to my office so that he could support Gabrielle in getting from my waiting room to her dentist to treat her excruciatingly painful tooth abscess. They tag-teamed to ensure that Britney could still have her regular therapy session, even in the context of Gabrielle's health crisis. In the couple therapy sessions surrounding this event, they spoke about the way Maddox reached out lovingly to Gabrielle and the way she accepted his support, rather than rejecting him, as she used to do. In Britney's individual sessions and her parents' couple sessions, we discussed how she had felt deeply supported by her parents as a loving couple committed to preserving her therapy. This experience resulted from sessions in which we analysed the ways the couple lapsed into archaic and destructive patterns of misperceiving one another as transference objects. Time and time again, we metabolised previously unconscious links that existed between Gabrielle and Maddox within the analytic field—links that had hitherto caused a serious impasse between them.

A later house built by Britney provided a testament to the growth of the family's interpersonal unconscious (Figure 10.3). The inside and outside of the house became more distinguishable, by her repositioning the tree to the outside, and bordering the front door with walls and flowers. She created more potential living spaces, with a kitchen, dining room, living room, TV room, hallway and entryway. The parents' master bedroom became entirely demarcated from the children's bedrooms. In sum, she represented her family's mind as more dynamic, organized, and structured.

Reflections

Looking back, complementing Britney's individual therapy with couple therapy for her parents resulted in a deepening of her therapy and contributed to

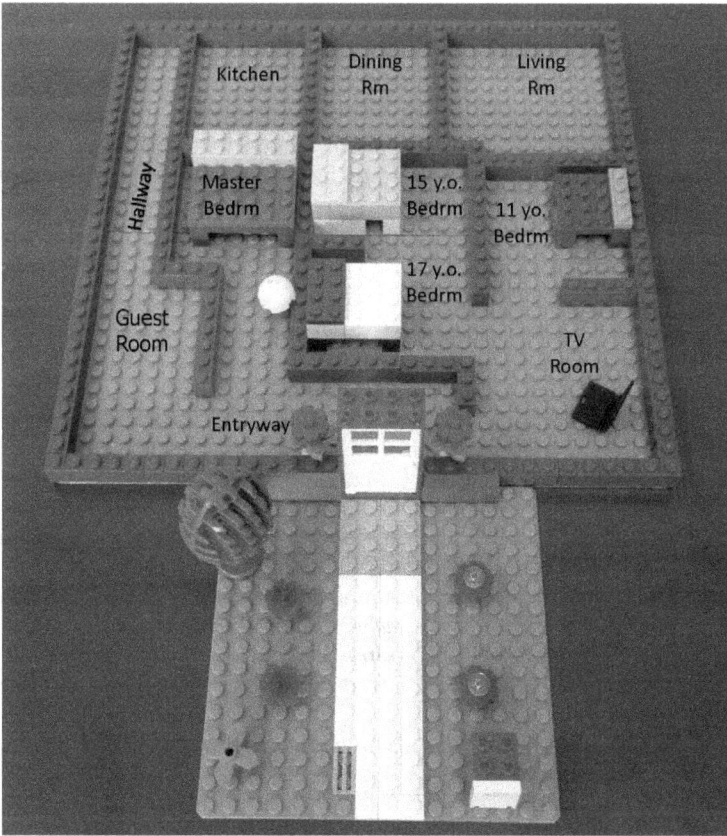

Figure 10.3 Later iteration of Britney's Lego house

a marked improvement in her symptoms and adaptation to her life both inside and outside the family. Gabrielle and Maddox were then more able to bring their previously unspoken traumas into the room to be verbalised and reflected upon, rather than perpetually re-enacted. As their marriage has stabilised, they have been more able to provide a container for each other and for their children; Accordingly, they became less apt to project their aggression and heightened sexual longings into their children. Furthermore, they became able to recognize their son's needs, and hence access a therapy for him.

This therapeutic strategy of conjoint individual and couple therapy helped the family move beyond the impasses that brought them to therapy. It took much more analytic child and couple work before the "problematic ghosts of [their] represented past [could] be converted…to useful ancestors for the present" (Emde, 2005, p. 118). Link and field theories operate as organising frameworks to listen to the interpersonal unconscious, and to hold and integrate these separate therapy configurations. Analytic couple and family work inspires the hope that we can interrupt the further transmission of such links among current and future generations and can facilitate the creation of healthier links.

In closing, I would like to express my gratitude to Britney and her family who have enriched my clinical understanding of the applications of link and field theories, and to David and Jill Scharff for offering us a readable and in-depth discussion of link and field theories in *The Interpersonal Unconscious*.

References

Baranger, M. 2005. Field Theory. In: S. LewkowiczandS. Flechner (Eds), *Truth, Reality and the Psychoanalyst: Latin American Contributions to Psychoanalysis* (pp. 49–71). London: International Psychoanalytical Association.

Baranger, M. and Baranger, W. 1961/1962[2008]. The Analytic Situation as a Dynamic Field. *International Journal of Psycho-analysis*, 89: 795–825.

Bion, W. 1962. *Learning From Experience*. London: Heinemann.

Emde, R.N. 2005. A Developmental Orientation for Contemporary Psychoanalysis. In: G. Gabbard, E. Pearson and A. Cooper (Eds), *Textbook of Psychoanalysis* (pp. 117–130). Washington, DC: American Psychiatric Publishing.

Ferro, A. 2009. Transformations in Dreaming and Characters in the Psychoanalytic Field. *International Journal of Psychoanalysis*, 90: 209–230.

Pichon-Rivière, E. 1956/1957[1985]. *Teoría del vínculo, selección temática de transcripciones de sus clases, años 1956/57*, F. Taragano (Ed.). (1985). Buenos Aires: Nueva Visión.

Scharff, D.E. and Scharff, J.S. 2011. *The Interpersonal Unconscious*. Lanham, MD: Jason Aronson.

11 Cyberspace as Refuge or Prison: An Exploration of Analytic Communication

Majlis Winberg Salomonsson

Psychoanalysis changes over time. We refine the theoretical concepts, and the clinic is expanded to reach new patient groups. In society, modern technology makes it possible to communicate with each other in new ways. Psychoanalysis is usually described as "the talking cure". For this reason, we might regard letters, e-mail or other communication on the Internet as tending more towards the opposite, as a form of action. But the matter is not quite that simple. We need only remember that Freud's own self-analysis took place to a considerable extent in the form of correspondence with Wilhelm Fliess via letters. When he analysed Marie Bonaparte, they read together from her diaries, which she brought along to her analysis sessions.

In our analytic work, all of us have met the new communication via Internet, which has downright exploded in recent years. This is a phenomenon that has come to stay. Information technology is described as the fourth communication revolution. The first was the spoken word, the second the written word and the third the printed word. Young people today use Internet daily. It has been found that most young people communicate online with their family, their friends, and others they already know (Dunkels et al., 2011). In other words, young Internet users who contact people they do not know constitute a small group. They are at great risk of running into serious harm through contacts online, contacts which can lead to various forms of crime, including sexual exploitation.

In our work, the new technology can have special consequences. Some time ago I met a teenage girl who wanted me to go to her blog to find out more about her. It turned out she had, not *one* blog, she had *three*. So, if I had gone along with this request, I would have been spending not only four hours of analysis per week on her but full time. Moreover, I would have got to know just one version of her, and it would not be a real communication between the two of us. One of my analysands said: "E-mail is a direct line to you - always!" We could say that in this way she wanted to put the framework of psychoanalysis out of play, the framework that says that we meet at certain times, that there are limitations for our contact.

DOI: 10.4324/9781003246749-11

There are some things that the patient finds much more difficult to say in words face-to-face than to write about in an e-mail or blog or on Facebook. These difficulties most often concern feelings: falling in love, sex, anger, and hatred. It can be easier to tell your analyst what you feel when sitting at home in front of the computer than when you are in the analytic session. We could say that from the patient's perspective, conveying something in writing via Internet provides a kind of privacy, a chance to avoid the analytic expectation to associate freely during the analysis session and to go into mutual communication with the analyst.

A special aspect of e-mail is that many people feel that it frees them from responsibility. When they send the e-mail, it is out there. Glenn Gabbard (2001) has written about his work with an analysand who used her e-mail to communicate her strong sexual attraction to her analyst. She said of her e-mail messages: "They are out there, and they have already been sent. I no longer have any responsibility for them." Gabbard describes how he in his countertransference could feel the enticement and desire to enter a mutual understanding with his analysand via e-mail communication. They could be out there together in cyberspace, and nobody else would know.

The communication between two people sitting at their computers, each at a different location, is not actually *inside* the world but it is not *outside* either. We find here an intermediate area, which is interesting to explore. This is where the concept of cyberspace comes in. How can we then define cyberspace? The term has roots in the Greek *kybernetes*, which means something like helmsman, pilot or rudder and was first used by a science fiction writer, William Gibson.

We can make a comparison with the telephone: Cyberspace is the place where the telephone call is going on. The call is not inside the telephone, the device we hold in our hand, nor in the other person's telephone. It is in the space between the telephones, this electrical space, the link that goes from the one telephone to the other. Since the 1960s the telephone has been expanded with computers and television and although we cannot speak of a physical place, we can describe cyberspace in terms of space.

So, what is happening out there on the net? People communicate with each other, obtain information, play games, and build up entire communities (second life). For example, people can fall head over heels in love with each other on the Internet without having met at all.

What distinguishes this virtual reality from the inner world and from external reality? And what kind of implications does this virtual reality have for the relation between the analyst and the patient. Virtual reality is not the same as the fantasy life of the inner world, nor the same as the tangible physical presence of outer reality.

The very concept of virtual reality can be traced to a French poet, playwright and theatre director Antonin Artaud. In his book from 1938, *The Theatre and Its Double*, he describes theatre as "la réalite virtuelle". The theatre shows something that is not real, it is fiction. What Artaud said is also true of the virtual reality that we encounter today. Many people who live large parts of their lives online can be tempted to mix up virtual reality and actual reality. Virtual reality is what I would call an illusion. Not everyone agrees with me. Both Internet users and some researchers would say instead that virtual reality is another reality. They speak about "in virtual life" as opposed to "in real life".

Youth of today live sizeable portions of their lives at the computer. Young people are out on Facebook, MSN or YouTube, they chat, they play games, and they work at the computer. They can choose and change their identity when they are online, their name, their age, their gender and so forth. This can function as a place to experiment with different identities.

Jonathan was one of these boys who played games on their own when he came to my clinic for the first time. He was completely encapsulated in his own world at the computer. It took years of analytic work to obtain a picture of the content of his cyberworld, what it meant for him and to explore and discover what it would take to convince him to go leave his enclosed world and communicate with others in real life.

Jonathan's parents got in contact with me when he is fourteen years old. He frequently sat quite alone at the computer in his room and seldom came out to take part in family activities. Several years earlier, at the onset of puberty, Jonathan stayed home from school more and more and during the last two years, he had only been at school sporadically. All efforts to help him to return to school have failed because of the agitation and intense resistance awakened in him. When the family first came to me, Jonathan had been formally assigned to private teaching, in which he seldom participated. His mother and the school counsellor were deeply concerned about the situation, from the standpoints of his well-being and of uncertainty about the future.

His mother was worried that Jonathan had so few friends and had such a hard time keeping the ones he had made. Ever since he has been at home all the time, he has had no friends at all. He has never mentioned any contacts with girls, nor had any girls come for a visit. His mother was also concerned that Jonathan often stayed up late and, in those cases, sits mostly alone at the computer in his room. She has asked what he does there and has been told that he plays games online. He was also rather finicky and almost obsessive-compulsive about keeping order in his room. His father conveyed that his son seems to have a good head on his shoulders and is no doubt going to be fine. He was not especially worried that Jonathan stays at home. He thought Jonathan was good at computers and he pointed out that Jonathan was good at school, as long as he attended regularly. Jonathan himself seemed to have a hard time knowing what he wanted. He did not seem to want anything or to express any wishes. He did not directly express any need for help while at the same time he was not negative towards the idea of coming to therapy sessions. He gave no sign of feeling that anything was wrong.

The first time I met Jonathan I saw a quiet boy with a hint of a smile on his face. He settled down slowly in the chair, his medium-long hair hanging down and hiding a part of his face. He told me laconically how he stays in his room most of the time and plays games on his computer. He mentioned that he comes out to the family at mealtimes, at least sometimes. He thought that it is too bad that his friends did not get in touch with him so much these days. However, he did not have any regrets about not going to school. Towards the end of the session, he said that he is okay with coming to see me again, so we book some new appointments.

To talk to Jonatan about school, about the importance of going out and making social contacts, is futile. In this respect I am facing a wall. He is just smiling, avoids my interpretations, talks about something else or simply becomes silent. At first, I feel frustrated and look for other ways of communicating with him. Eventually I found that to learn something about the world that Jonathan has created with the help of computer games turns out to be both possible and important—and disquieting. As our sessions progress, I gradually get a glimpse into his life behind the closed door of a teenaged boy's room. Jonathan tells me more and more about how he constructs his own games online. He is eager to explain the approaches that he uses in creating his games. He gets excited in a way that I have never seen him before, quickly takes out a sketchbook and shows me how he does everything. For the first time I feel a real contact with him, that I am included.

So, what do the games look like? The games that Jonathan constructs follow the same pattern that we know so well. The main character makes his journey through perils of different kinds, through labyrinths and caves, encountering monsters and hideous beasts. He is equipped with various weapons and attributes, which can be picked up and lost during the journey. He can lose his life and regain it a certain number of times. An obvious feature of Jonathan's games is their degree of violence. He puts great emphasis on how terrifying his characters look and how gory a spectacle their battles become. A quiet, outwardly peaceful boy sits here in front of me but behind the closed door of his room he lives an entirely different life. He creates a world where violence rules, where war rages between beasts and humans and where sadism is prevalent. And—not least important—where he reigns supreme. Here at last is a place where he can be the one who decides. Here he is not the awkward boy who cannot cope with school, who fails at friendship and who has no girlfriend. Here he is master over life and death. This fantasy of superiority, this omniscient notion, took a long time to approach. This was a secret world that Jonathan allowed me to enter only after we had built up a sense of trust, a rapport, where he could believe in my genuine interest about how he was thinking and how things were going in his life.

Now I could also better understand how Jonathan was entrapped. How would he be able to gain the strength to leave this world that he had built up and where he was the king, yes, a king with absolute power, and instead venture out into a world where he would be at the mercy of others, where he did not know if the others would accept him, where he did not have control, where he felt vulnerable to others' whims, whether good or bad?

His caution and dread towards entering relationships, into contacts with others, became discernible in the sessions with me. I would like to give an example of how an analysis session at the beginning of our work could look:

Jonathan comes in and sits down in his chair. He has the hint of a smile on his face as usual. He says:

-The next issue of *Illustrated Science* is going to be about memory. They say that there are different centres in the brain for different memories.
-Mm…you are interested in the memory.
-Right, they say that the left part of the brain is more insensitive. Hm, that would mean that left-handed people should be more sensitive. But that's not true in my case. I never cry when I go to the cinema. And I am not very sensitive to pain either.

There are a few moments of silence. He looks around and catches sight of a book on my bookshelf:

-Aha, *Åke and his World*. So, it's obviously about a boy and how he views the world.
-You think so?
-Yes, that would fit in here, you know. (He lets out a little laugh and continues.) I recognise the title, but I don't remember.
-Mm…memory again.
-Right, whenever I want to know something, I check it out online.
-And when there's something you can't find out online?
-Well, then I wait and see…
-You wait?
-Yes, or maybe I'm not so interested in it anyway, so…
-Hm, I wonder about that…
-Okay, maybe not always but it's easier when I can check it out online.
-Yes, because then you don't need to ask anyone. You don't need to show others that you don't know. After all, it can be hard to do that.

There is another silence. We hear a sound from the street. Jonathan says:

-It sounds like the air raid alarm. Are they testing it today?

He continues for a moment to think aloud about how they test the alarm, which days they usually do it, whether it is every week or only once a month, and so forth.

I say:

> -Well, there was an alarm now. Maybe it became an alarm for you when we were talking about you and what you show to others. Maybe it's not so easy to show things here either.

He starts to talk about an alarm that went off on the street where he lives one time when he was little, around six or seven years old. There was a fire in the bakery near his house. The plume of smoke was high, "it was so high that you couldn't see where it ended." When I ask what he thought about that, he says, "It was awesome."

I say:

> -So you would rather go on talking about alarms than talk about the things I mentioned?

He smiles:

> -Yep!

Jonathan sits there looking around. His gaze returns to my bookshelf. A book catches his attention.

> -*The Interpretation of Dreams*. Aha, dreams. And to think that I didn't dream anything last night either. It seems like I dream less now since I started in therapy.
> -Mm. It seems like now, when we would be able to talk about your dreams, well, they go into hiding. That door is closed.
> -Well, two nights or so ago I had a dream, but I don't remember what it was about.

He tells me about a dream that he had when he was younger, when he was seven or eight years old or so:

> -I saw a meatball. It was an enormous meatball with a big fork in it. It was dark blue, in the evening or the night. There were mountains in the background, high mountains. And then I saw Anna (older sister) come riding along. She rode on the head of a big dinosaur.

When I ask him what he is thinking, he says that he likes meatballs.

When the session is over and he is getting ready to go out, he turns at the door and says:

> -Mm, it smells like food here.

The session gets under way with Jonathan talking about memory. I have heard about his interest in science several times. He speaks in detail about various measurable things and at the same time often gives the impression that this is his way of keeping something else at a distance, something that could engage him emotionally. He senses something threatening based on the article in *Illustrated Science* and underscores for me that all that stuff about the left part of the brain and sensitivity, as he has interpreted it, does not apply to him. Sensitive is something he is not.

Then a book on my bookshelf catches his eye, as has happened before. Of all the books on the shelves it is *Åke and his World* and *The Interpretation of Dreams* that his gaze falls upon. In both situations, he stakes out a certain distance. *Åke and his World*, well, that's something he would obviously expect to see here. Dream interpretation, well, he has not had any dreams, especially not since he started analysis. In my countertransference, I can feel downgraded and placed a little on the outside of things, tricked. It is as if he is conveying to me: don't think you can just get access to my world as easily as that.

Jonathan says that when there is something that he wants to know, he checks online. Based on my feeling of being made an outsider by him, I suggest that he goes online but does not seek contact with people. I was no doubt right basically, but he could not take in this comment. His inner being sets off an alarm and I comment on that. The defence interpretation works, and it is here that we can meet in mutual communication.

So, to the interpretation of dreams. Jonathan has admitted earlier that he finds it an interesting phenomenon. But with a certain degree of triumph, he can assert that he has no dreams to offer, at least not from his present life situation. He tells me about a dream that he had when he was around seven or eight years old. That was a long time ago and he does not have the same responsibility today for the dreams he had as a child since he was so young after all. So, what can we do with this material here and now? We can agree that it is about food, an enormous meatball, a kind of food that he likes. The comment he makes as he is leaving is clearly positive. He is now clearly more positive to the analysis situation, and to me. But the meatball was attacked with a fork. I could sense that he dared to approach me. Obviously, strong aggressive and destructive impulses are also involved here.

Jonathan seems to be struggling with the thought of entering into a relationship with me and at the same time maintaining his customary distance, the same way he acts towards most of the people and things around him.

What then would get Jonathan to leave this splendid isolation? Ultimately, it is going to be profoundly lonely in there. It can be said that the world that Jonathan created online did not represent freedom at all. Maybe it felt like some kind of liberation in the beginning, a breathing space when anxiety became too strong and when he had a hard time enduring his ordinary external life. But this fortress of freedom was soon transformed into a prison, a prison where he admittedly had power, but where he also was completely alone. Through the way he told me about his games, about how he constructed them and how he created various strategies for playing them, we could explore together how he had built up an inner universe. It took a long time for him to develop a trust in me, to confide to me glimpses of this world and an even longer time for him to be ready for a change.

Here are some details from another session with Jonathan about one year later. He has now started to attend a special class at school.

As soon as Jonathan has entered the analysis room, he says immediately:

-From today it is sixteen days until I come here again.
-Yes, you are keeping a careful check.
-Right, you are cancelling next week. And tomorrow as well.
-Mm…
-Why?

He looks straight at me, smiling slightly.

-That was a good question. Maybe you wonder what I am going to be doing.
-Hm…

I realise that I do not really understand him correctly, so I say:

-Or maybe you mean that I should not have cancelled so many sessions.
-Yep.
-So that is what you want to say, that you do not like it at all.
-Precisely.
-OK, I can understand that. I give myself rights like this and just cancel your sessions.
-Mm.

We talk about how various things that concern him are simply decided upon and he does not know so much about why… It is like this at school for example, he says. When I wonder what he does in case there is something he wants to know or ask about, he says that they probably cannot give him an answer anyway. Or he just waits and sees. But, I say, you did not do so today. Here he showed me what he thought. And he asked.

Jonathan tells me that today he succeeded at diving into the deep-water swimming pool for the first time. He has known for several years from a strictly theoretical standpoint what he should do with his ears to adjust to the pressure so that he can go deeper but today was the first time that he could actually do it. He went all the way to the bottom, 4 ½ meters! It was awesome, he says.

I comment that he dared. I add that we can speak of daring to dive into the pool, and we can also speak of daring to say things here with me in analysis.

He starts to talk about a boy in his class who has shown him a new computer game that he had. He says:

-It was super. I'd like to get one like that.

For the first time in analysis, he tells me about a dream he has just had:

-I dreamed last night. I was going to eat a pizza. I was going to test which one was best, the pizzeria near my home or the one on the corner near here. Then I woke up.

When I wonder what he is thinking, he does not know. I say:

-You are dreaming about home and about here. It seems as if you are comparing: what can you get there at home and what can you get here?

At this point he starts talking about the book *The Hitchhiker's Guide to the Galaxy*. He tells me that in that book they ask a question about meaning and the computer finally answers: 42. But how should you ask the question and what is the question and what does the answer mean? He tells me that what happens in the book is that the earth, which is just one giant computer, and which was just about to be able to ask the question, explodes the second before anyone gets to know anything. I comment that it seems to be a matter of impossible questions and impossible answers, and nobody gets to know. He smiles and says:

-Right, you got it.

Even so, these are no doubt questions that are important for him, I comment. He sighs and says:

-Yes, that's the way it is.

Jonathan begins the session with an emotionally charged message. He presents it like a fact with an exactness that almost gives an obsessive-compulsive impression. He counts the days, as if this act of counting the exact number of days is more important than the emotional content. Are 16 days a long or short time? My first comment stems from my guess that he might be wondering about me as a person, about what I am going to be doing during those cancelled sessions. But it turns out that he is pre-occupied with the thought that I am not going to be here, not under his control, that I am going to be doing my own things and thus putting him in a vulnerable position. Usually in his effort to process such difficult feelings, he says something such as he does not care; it makes no difference to him. Here he comes out with another reaction, albeit not immediately, but with all clarity after a comment from me. He shows me that he is vulnerable and that something is missing when I am not there.

I make it a point to stress this to him: that he actually questioned me about my cancellations. He did not just wait. My assertion leads him to tell me about an initiative that he took at the swimming pool. He had figured out how to dive! He had dared and succeeded. I could not help but draw a parallel to our work in analysis, to dive down. Jonathan seemed to accept this. He goes on and talks about new ventures that might be possible to take on.

In this session we see his struggle between interacting with the world outside and entering into a relationship versus staying in his own splendid isolation. It seems perilous to get to know, to find out things, not least things about his inner world. But now he shows that he wants to learn things, or perhaps we should say, he wants to know things, to know how to do things.

A new sense of trust has come into being. To tell about a recent dream is for Jonathan a truly dare-devilish undertaking. It means that he is exposing something about himself without knowing what it is or what is going to become of it. Or what I will be able to make of it! He has shared a confidence with me, and I feel that I must take wise care of it. The ordinary work with dream associations and so forth is not possible to carry out. I can however hold onto the insight that he is preoccupied with thoughts of how it is to be at home and how it is to be in analysis, thoughts about relating to me, that is to say, to direct himself outward towards the object. Even this sequence concerns food. The regressive or perhaps we should say the basal, the primal needs, are in focus. Where can nourishment be found? Is it possible to get sustenance here? The questions are many and the answers are still unknown. Jonathan gives a powerful analogy for this dilemma by mentioning the example from *The Hitchhiker's Guide to the Galaxy*, an almost surrealistic vision of the future.

Things gradually begin to happen behind the closed door, both metaphorically speaking in Jonathan's inner being and literally in his external world. Jonathan begins to dare to show more of who he is in his communication with me, what he wants and what he fears. At home in his room, he starts to take contact with others on the Internet and starts to join in games together with others. There was a feeling of uncertainty in the beginning of his analysis. It all felt so risky for him. Now he had started to take part in games where he did not have control over the rules. He gained respect from others, he found acknowledgement that he knew a great deal, but he has also had to meet competition. There were others who knew more than he did.

Jonathan used the computer and his self-constructed games over a long period of time to build up a secret world of his own, a world where he acted out his sadistic fantasies and where time stood still. In these games he created his own identity. It was partly his own self, but it was not all of him! Major parts of it were a false identity! He created an illusion about the world. His world on the computer was completely his own. He did not address himself to anyone else, not even in the virtual world. Through analysis, when he dared more and more to enter relationships with others, he could also change his game routines and get into contact with other like-minded gamers online.

We can ask ourselves the question: Is the communication of computers in the virtual world an aid for human communication? Are there risks and what is the nature of the risks? Does this communication change us to the core or does it accentuate certain sides of our personality? Communication in the virtual world has more to do with the accumulation of knowledge and with performance than with feelings or the development of the thinking that arises from this communication. The virtual world has an entirely different relationship to the lust principle and the reality principle than do both the inner and the outer word. The virtual world gives an *illusion* of what is real, as if the computer user would not need to mentally process the link between the inner world and the outer reality. The readymade images in virtual reality then become pseudo-representations of pseudo-objects. In this way, the relationship to the computer user's inner world become unclear. All this leads to a notion that it is actually not important to develop any inner communication. For this reason, it would be interesting to explore further what is happening in the link between symbolisation, which is of course a three-dimensional relationship, and the artificial intelligence in the virtual world, which is a two-dimensional relationship.

Virtual communication in the computer world entails risks on the individual level for our analytic work. Florence Guignard (in her presentation at European Psychoanalytic Federation, 2009) has emphasised primarily two risks: an expectation for instantaneous realisation of wishes and desires, on the model of what happens in a virtual world and an increased risk that basic assumption group mentality (Bion, 1961) will take over from thinking for oneself.

My experiences of work with young people, who spend their time online daily, have shown me that their computer use can take on many different forms. Jonathan tried to satisfy his desire for omnipotence by creating his own autocracy in computer games, an illusion that he clung onto stubbornly for several years. His entry into this world coincided with the onset of puberty. It gradually became clearer and clearer that his desire for control also had to do with dread in the face of drive impulses, both sexual and aggressive, that had started to manifest themselves. He got an outlet for unarticulated needs in these self-constructed games as a substitute for in relations to others.

We can have cause to be observant as to how our analysands use computers, how they communicate online and how they contact us via e-mail and so on. Does the communication take place as an attempt to put the analytic framework out of play, to deny time, yes, when taken to the ultimate extreme, to deny death? Or does it take place to exchange information, to obtain knowledge?

My work with Jonathan illustrates the importance of examining the virtual scenarios that our analysands show us. Here we return to the question of inner or outer objects in cyberspace. Or is it rather a question of inanimate objects? In that case analytic work needs to be directed so that these inanimate objects are given life, that they are transformed into emotional representations and do not remain processes that are evacuated or acted out.

In other words, we need to focus our interest not only on the outer technical consequences of Internet but also on what the use of the Internet means for the inner world. That is to say, we need to take it into the analytic conversation and examine it with our analytic method.

References

Artaud, A. 1938. *The Theatre and Its Double*. London, Alma Classics.

Bion W.R. 1961. *Experiences in Groups and Other Papers*. London, Tavistock.

Dunkels, E., Frånberg, G-M. and Hällgren, C. 2011. *Youth culture and net culture: Online social Practices*. New York.

Gabbard, G. 2001. Cyberpassion: E-Rotic Transference on the Internet, *Psychoanal. Quarterly*, 70(4): 719–737.

Guignard, F. 2009. Transformation of instincts in digital and in symbolic mental functioning: the future of oblivion. Paper at the European Psychoanalytic Federation.

12 New Voices in Child Analysis

Autistic functioning and psychic pain? Building up possible links

Mariângela Mendes de Almeida

Introduction: A dyad at risk?

Psychoanalytic work with autistic states, either in children with autistic disorders or in our daily contact with the autistic enclaves of our non-autistic patients, has represented a creative and fruitful challenge to the development of our clinical field. It has expanded the range of our eyes and ears to nonverbal communication, including subtle signs of contact and distance regulation between patient and analyst. It has, therefore, fostered the discussion and development of clinical tools for accessing primitive states of mind.

Working with children and infants at risk within the context of their initial relationships has also broadened and deepened basic psycho-analytic conceptualisations to include the fertilising interface with clinical and research developments within psychoanalytic infant observation, child psychology and neurosciences (Alvarez, 1992; Stern, 1985; Trevarthen, 2011). Contemporary psychoanalytic developments in which countertransference constitutes a privileged tool to access psychic quality in our patients and in ourselves has nurtured our professional practice and clinical discussions (Ferro, 1995; Barros, 2008, 2009, 2011; Spessoto, 2009).

Autistic states and psychic pain? Is this a feasible dyad to work with? Or, is this a dyad at risk of non-integration and non-existence? Is autistic func-tioning not a possible and effective defence/shielding against any awareness of psychic suffering and separation between the self and other? The usual working through psychic pain, developed as one of the core elements of our psychoanalytic practice, does not take place in the same way within this primitive area. The intersubjective relationship needs to be constructed and the analyst needs to recognise and contain the specific shape of transfers (Ferro, 1995) within a no- or nearly-object relation (Alvarez, 1992) rather than the classic object related transference.

As a metaphor, this conceptual dyad—autistic states and psychic pain—might be seen as a dyad at risk, in need of some "early intervention" considering both sides in their detailed interaction. As with the

DOI: 10.4324/9781003246749-12

intersubjective relationship between an autistic child and his caregiver, the relationship between autistic states and psychic pain might not exist—it needs to be constructed as part of the psychoanalytic treatment. This dyad, with its peculiar nuances, is also at risk of not being carefully examined, even within our own "psychoanalytic family". As an example, I was recently approached by a senior colleague, with great psychoanalytic experience with adult neurotic patients, while I was preparing a video for a presentation of an autistic patient treated for eight years. The video starts with domestic scenes of the four-year-old patient, in which there is no language or communication, no interpersonal look or shared attention, with clear signs of intense withdrawal and attraction to the sensorial quality of the experience. There are also scenes showing the psycho-analytic work with the patient and the multidisciplinary approach offered to him in a therapeutic school. The video ends with the patient (then aged 12) "interviewed" by professionals in regular contact with him, and shows verbal language, narratively organised in attuned responses. Although his vocal tone and articulation are a somewhat rigid and stiff, the patient refers to himself, to his family and makes spontaneous comments about friends at school. My experienced colleague watched the video, and then commented: "He was not autistic, then!" Over the course of the decades-long tradition of working with autistic states, this is, unfortunately an all too common experience for colleagues working in the field. Paradoxically, conceptual contributions arising from this field have been found useful and fruitful to general psychoanalytic development, such as Tustin's con-cepts of autistic objects and shapes and autistic aspects in neurotic patients (1981), and Meltzer's ideas about dimensionalities (1975).

Coming back to the dyad at risk, if, on the one hand, autistic function-ing contains a difficulty in allowing contact with psychic pain or lacks the mental apparatus to acknowledge and work through it; on the other hand, the analyst, as well as the child's parents/family, experience the most extreme feelings of despair, hopelessness, dissolution, non-existence and loneliness. Psychoanalytic interventions are certainly more consistent when considering our psychic pain through a refined work with our countertransference and through including the possibility of containing parental psychic suffering along with our treatment with the child.

Clinical background: current dimensions

The intense anxieties experienced by an autistic child's family members and professional network are understandable when the continuity and gradual spiral of interactive and dialogic exchanges remain unnourished by the difficulty in sustaining communicative and emotional responses. The analytic function implies empathy with the psychic pain suffered by caregivers from the absence or loss of aspects that are as banal as they are essential cornerstones of child development, like not looking, seeming not to hear, having no interest in playing or shows of affection, and self-imposed isolation.

Contemporary clinical and conceptual thinking discusses the analyst's mental activity towards the patient as a live and active invitation to contact (the "reclamation" in the "live company" referred by Anne Alvarez, 1992) based on incipient rudiments of interest, proto-bonding elements whose relational content strengthens with the analyst's emotional drive addressing the subject and deeply investing in building up a link with the patient (Marucco, 2007; Mendes de Almeida, 2008; Silva, Mendes de Almeida and Barros, 2011). Expanding this context to the broader scope of caregiving (family and educational contexts), analysts often see themselves trying to maintain alive, acknowledge, rescue, return, restore and strengthen the investments by caregivers in emotional and developmental links—investments so threatened by being weakened that they can, sometimes, even be extinguished.

Offering containment and holding for parental anxieties in integration with the child's analytic process has been supported by developments in psychoanalytic theory and techniques (Alvarez and Reid, 1999; Laznik, 1995; Sherkow, 2008), informed by the contributions of Stern (1985) and Trevarthen (2011) in the fields of child development, psychoanalytic observation of the parent-infant relationship and its unfolding by Williams and Mélega (Sonzogno and Mélega, 2008), therapeutic consultation by Winnicott and its applications by Lebovici (1983, 1986), joint interventions in initial relationships (Mélega and Mendes de Almeida, 2007; Mendes de Almeida, Marconato, Silva, 2004; Silva, 2002), along with the questioning of the traditional technique of (not) working with the parents over the course of a classic child analytic process (Lisondo et al., 1996).

Whether in joint parent-child sessions or in regular contact between the child's parents and analyst when the child is seen individually, parents are currently seen with less worry of harmful interferences to the analytic setting, as potential and structural agents in the building up of emotional links. The analyst might also be available to link the surrounding support network or connect to institutions/professionals responsible for care, as well as communicating his psychoanalytic comprehension, as shown below.

This construction also involves expanding the child's and parents' contact with the experience of psychic pain - i.e. an increase in the degree of experiencing emotional states (Bion's learning from emotional experience, 1962), allowing movements in the continuum between states of non-integration and integration as a founding part of human development. These movements might go from the natural primitive states of non-integration and, if not finding containment, regulation and modulation in the psychic environment of parental care, might condense into nameless dread, catastrophic anxiety, fear of collapse, states of dissolution, liquefaction and annihilation anxiety. However, there might be also experiences of possibly integrate psychic pain and suffering, even if in rudimentary representations: there are many wefts to weave into the work with autistic disorders.

Regarding the possibility of a genuine inclusion of children with autistic disorders in schools and social circles, it is important to emphasise the integrating character of the inclusion of the analytic point of view to their families and educators. If, on the one hand, the entry of the analyst can provide new constructs, it can also, on the other hand, be presented as disruptive to "routines" (including psychic ones) established as part of a "protective homeostasis" when facing emotional suffering.

These aspects are illustrated below in the case of a young child undergoing analysis where we can see seminal issues of the establishment of a mind with the ability to tolerate states of emotional diversity and plasticity, including experiences of discontinuity that can (or not) come to be represented and felt as psychic pain.

Patrick, his parents and the constitution of a network of containment

Patrick begins analysis at the age of three years, one month: a child with clear autistic functioning and parents expectantly awaiting the start of an analytic process after receiving assessment.

The child had been referred by his speech therapist (who he sees twice a week, owing to his speech delay) to a psychiatrist (also an analyst), who brought up the child's situation and the need for analytic treatment.

Mother makes contact immediately, and the parents come for a session, including themselves and the other professionals (speech therapist, teachers, psychoanalyst), as part of a "task force" to tackle Patrick's autism. They mention that, perhaps owing to Patrick being an only child, they remained unaware of his difficulties, considering them as normal development (it was "all so cute"). They feel resentful for not having been alerted earlier, at their initial paediatric consultations.

Besides Patrick's delay in starting to talk, they emphasise his difficulty in leaving behind the nappy and baby bottle, an intense and anxious contact with certain objects (some books, videos and a baby blanket), and a determined grinding of his teeth.

They bring a large envelope and express their bewilderment, owing to the fact that all the exam results are normal (Guthrie test, brain scan, audiometric exams, amino acid chromatographic exam), yet the definitive diagnosis now seems to be Autistic Disorder. Patrick goes to a normal nursery, full-time during the week.

In the beginning, Patrick and his parents come for joint sessions, followed by some individual, exploratory sessions. After that, we began a process of three sessions a week with Patrick and one session a month with his parents.

Managing nappies and bottles: from discomfort-placating "pacifiers" to the possibility of regulation and modulation

Since the beginning, Patrick's expression of "expectancy" is very noticeable. His eyes are wide open, suggesting a contact without mediation or modulation that at times seems frightened, at others, distant, far away, directed at a "supposed" void. Sometimes, however, it seems connected, even if fleetingly and elusively. Sad? Suffering? Patrick cries out as if he is "feeling something", perhaps intriguingly not just desperately evacuating unprocessable contents. What "psychic meaning" can we find in his upset crying? Is it my feeling or his feeling that is counter-transferentially felt? His facial expressions and emotional atmosphere flicker within seconds. He can go from being apparently calm and involved, to suddenly seeming irritated and reacting with abrupt movements, or interrupting a wave of irritation with a sudden smile (at times more connected, at others less, with jumpy movements, looking at his own hand as it moves delicately in front of and above his face).

Much of his expression comes from his breathing sounds, laleos, variations in the issuing of sounds, sometimes whispered, sometimes guttural manifestations that I associate with the repertoire of a baby in contact with his primary care figures, and that I have tried to amplify in a relational context. Here, it is interesting to think about the threshold between ritualization and autistic manifestation versus the child's exploration of sounds and the seeds of communication.

The teeth grinding is, in fact, surprising and even with his mouth closed, the rhythmic tension still echoes around the room. What would be the boundaries between a prospective experience of psychic pain that has not yet arisen and the discomfort of a sensorial experience of excitation, overloading and tension involved in states of shielding and physical armouring to face a threat of collapse and imminent dissolution? This somatopsychic experience cannot yet be represented; it has neither figurability nor "thinkability" as a feeling to be communicated to other people around, through shareable language or expression. The analyst's mind and presence are needed as a bridge to build up that possible route.

There are times when the grinding only fully disappears when interspersed with bouts of crying whose meanings do not yet seem accessible. His entire body becomes entirely slack, his defences (are they defences?) are lowered and his silence or bizarre sounds are replaced by powerful weeping. This is apparently directed at something (someone?), leading something (from himself?), running through his "soma", appearing to lightly pass through his "psyche", but often being intercepted by a sudden interruption, or internal (dis)solution. These swings have been the subject of our "chats" during our sessions.

We weave ourselves through the analytic narrative and constant naming of situations, people and states; a "going on being" and continuing to be the same, despite the unexpected variations that, even if they still do not constitute suffering or psychic pains, configure themselves as disruptions that assault his sense of cohesion.

Much of our initial work takes place in the context of parent-child care and in connection with the health and education professionals involved. Patrick wears nappies during the initial sessions. I note that this large, strong and healthy lad sometimes seems to notice and be bothered by something "extra" on his body (the nappy in the summer heat). According to Patrick's parents at the time, he gives no sign before urinating or excreting, and always wears a nappy. His parents recognise the signs (as external products) after he begins. It seems that they, too, are "protected" by the "nappy" of the constant nappy routine. As the signs are very incipient, they do not correspond to the need for autonomy and expected signalisation. There is a tendency toward the crystallisation of an attitude of not acknowledging corporal needs and not communicating corporal events beyond themselves. Such events are not, therefore, characterised as arising from a body given meaning to by the gaze of the other/caregiver, which could establish a circuit of creating a subject. Fewer signs (or at least, very subtle ones), reduced communication, even less differentiation and ever more crystallisation characterise a vicious circle, both in this particular case of bladder and sphincter control, but also in the thinking about this situation for other areas of development.

Here, the interfaces that are so significant between the psychological aspects and the baby's or young child's somatic expressions are dramatically evident. They form the primary matrix for the way that discomforts can be felt, perceived, given meaning to and registered as a mark of the self, based upon the gaze of the other.

In this context, the psychoanalyst can help parents and other professionals to increase their observational acuity and sustain their belief that the chances of discrimination and subjectification will not die out. Integrating daily life with the possible universe of an aspiring psychic life, we agreed that Patrick would go without a nappy during the psychoanalytic sessions and visit the loo before starting. If there were any signs of discomfort or if he began to urinate or defecate, we would quickly take him to the bathroom, taking it as an opportunity to integrate his signs with attuned acknowledgement, physical manifestations with verbal language, and somatic with emotional experience.

The trips to the bathroom that follow, during the sessions, demonstrate the possibility of Patrick gradually recognising his internal needs, although they are interspersed with a few mishaps. One of these instances, which turned out to be messier and more uncontrolled than usual, was also especially embarrassing (agonising and painful!) for Patrick's father. Our analytic ability to metabolise and tolerate these aspects of a lack of control and deal with them as a necessary part of a transitional journey is important to avoid holding the parents to blame. It also allows the efforts to continue even in a vulnerable context - an aspect that often appears to underlie reduced investment, discredit and despair in disorders so destructive to intersubjectivity as autistic ones.

However, "protected" not (only) by the nappy, but also by the analytic setting and containing look, Patrick and his parents are able to establish a communication and sensitivity to the signs of need, with Patrick himself even being able to articulate the beginnings of the sound "pee". They demonstrate the ability to construct alternative devices for containment and regulation of flows between inside and outside, between self and other, and to make use of internal and relational psychic wrappings (the parents and child's bond with the analyst, the analyst's and parents' investment in the child's subjectivity, the child's recognition of his internal signs and the interest in communicating these signs to others, culminating with the possibility of developing bladder and bowel control).

Distress and the course of somatic discomfort gain new meaning within the realm of a possible communication of a state from oneself to another receptor and provider of care, one that is significant and brings transformation and reduced tension. These are ordinary paths in regular development, but in autistic functioning it might occur automatically, detached from emotional relationships. With Patrick and his parents, the previous homeostasis ensured by the means of repetition, stereotypes, automated routines and the terror of frustration, arrives now via an alternative path.

The proposed leaving behind of the nappy and its development is transmitted to the speech therapist and school during telephone and face to face conversations, but also at the initiative of the parents, who feel more confident in pursuing its course. The issue of the baby bottle and milk cup is also handled similarly in contact with the school. In the beginning, Patrick would always take a bottle to school, with his teachers feeling uncomfortable about taking it off him as he is always allowed it at home.

With his parents' increased capacity for containment, which is favoured by the care network strengthened by the analytic view, they feel more able to receive and transform Patrick's reactions of intolerance to change and insistence on maintaining sameness, known aspects of autistic disorders. (With understandable, yet risky relapses, such as being unable to prevent Patrick from carrying a large, round china plate with him wherever he went, and for which he maintained a ritualistic obsession for a time.)

On a visit to Patrick's school, I see that the teachers feel encouraged to substitute his bottle for the same kind of cup the other children use. I discuss Patrick, his advances and difficulties with his coordinator and class teacher. During snack time, he remains in his seat for less time than most of the other children, demonstrating no interest in eating and showing no attraction to the news that the teacher and teaching assistants enthusiastically and affectionately present.

Real inclusion seems threatened, with Patrick spoken about as someone who is restless and therefore needs to leave whenever the others congregate.

The bottle is something that keeps him together, "calm", with no apparent "suffering" (for him and for the others), but only supposedly and artificially, rather than symbolically included (Mendes de Almeida, 2004). The possibility of substituting the bottle, a facilitating element for keeping him "in the group", will be more feasible when both Patrick and his caregivers can count with more points of view and more care and comprehension alternatives, including the belief that he has the capacity to tolerate a process of change and separation from the conditions of fusion and non-differentiation.

These disruptions, initially and understandably experienced as very difficult by the caregivers and parents, can only be made in a genuine and incorporated manner, when they themselves can believe in their own capacity to tolerate these changes as well, and feel strengthened in the new containment alternatives on offer. This aspect illustrates how autistic rituals appear "comforting" in a certain way, as well as how the entry of an analyst can be disruptive and integrating at the same time.

Mirages and possibilities in the analytic scene

We have seen how the contact between parents and professionals, and among the professionals (school, speech therapist, analyst) are essential to creating a network in tune with the basic situations for the development of a young child like Patrick, where the interfaces between the physical and mental are so fundamentally interconnected. Habits from daily life might be integrated with psychic growth, including the possibility of glimpsing some of the child's tolerance to psychic discomfort and his need for meaning.

Below is a small excerpt from the end of a session where such issues manifest themselves more directly in the analytic scene:

> … Patrick picks up the plasticine, in which he had previously shown little interest. (He crumbled some between his fingers and then soon forgot about it.) Now, he seems more interested in it and wants to eat it. Using gestures, he "asks" me to remove the plastic wrap covering the plasticine. He picks up larger lumps and manipulates them with more consistency. I make "cakes" with the plasticine. A ball of plasticine rolls onto the floor and Patrick follows its route, sees where it gets to and goes to pick it up. (This is different from his previous indifference and lack of continuity in similar situations.) I mention to him how he followed the ball, saw where it went and brought it back for us to play with.
>
> (*I relate this with a sense of agency and continuity in the development of his intentions and wishes.*)

Patrick picks out smaller pieces, more jagged than the balls, but which are also more consistent than before, and makes an accompanying "p p p p" noise. I pick up a toy pan and put some of the small pieces inside it. Patrick watches me. He surreptitiously touches his shorts, near his bottom. Could this be a sign of his recognising a desire to poo? Or could it mean a less immediate association? I ask him if he wants to poo and make a comment about how now he knows that he has a feeling inside him like wanting to pee and wanting to poo that shows him that he wants to go to the bathroom. I say that he is becoming more aware of his desires and what he needs to do to make him feel better.

Patrick continues making the "p p p" sounds, which sometimes sound like "poo poo poo poo" and at others like "po po po po", but he does not move to go to the bathroom, as he has done before. Could he be relating in some other way (little ball, poo, something to do with his bottom, bathroom), to something more proto-representational? Could this be thought as a proto narrative, as in the beginnings of play? A mirage, or real possibilities?

Coming downstairs to meet his parents, Patrick is picked up by mother even before reaching the floor, straight from the stairway. This illustrates vividly how mother-child relationship still seems unable to support transitions, from being with a "caregiver"/analyst, then being able to be on his own, with his feet on the ground for a second, and then heading towards another "other".

The proposed parental modality for contact is still one of extension and continuity, it is still that of the mother-baby in arms, even in a situation where there seems to be the possibility of introducing small discontinuities and of walking under his own steam (of course, in motor terms this is possible, but is it psychically felt as such by the pair?). Our anticipation of this possibility is fundamental as a parental caregiver/container/investor element for our "baby" (the parents-child relationship itself), which begins being able to grow and take its steps. The analytic view of the child's and parents' potentials, rather than the automation committed to reducing immediate tensions, can introduce gradual breaches that help make flexible the emergence of unnamed terrors always waiting to strike. This might prevent spiralling anxiety, promoting a more stable condition to deal with changes, acknowledging and making use of ordinary, healthy abilities that, though present, are not always so evident.

Downstairs, just before leaving, the parents say that things are going well, but as Patrick was feeling somewhat under the weather, he went back to the bottle (The father says: "Her!" pointing to the mother as responsible, but in a tender way). They also say that he is still having difficulties with going number two in the toilet. Patrick always wants a nappy on to poo and ends up holding it in if no nappy is forthcoming. (The nappy ends up being put on him.)

I am interested by how the themes in the session and in the parents' accounts correspond and mention that Patrick also seems to be entrenched in the issue of perceiving his wills, recognising them and knowing when/

where he wants to go. They mention that things are fine when he wants to go number one, he warns them beforehand and has no problem using the toilet.

I wave goodbye to Patrick, who looks at me attentively. Whilst the mother leaves with Patrick in her arms, the father plays with them, waving goodbye to his son. Patrick looks at him with a serious and reproachful expression, an intense stare, and shakes his head "No" at the understood farewell given by the father. It is impossible to not feel, beyond a simple strangeness and a reaction to the break in sameness, the comprehension and evoking of a communication and of a proto-thinking, or a proto-mental process running its course in Patrick's mind! Could there be the beginnings of a space for noticing/being surprised/tolerating/feeling the separation and even housing in his mind-under-construction the doubt - will he come with us or not? Or, perhaps at this stage, is it simply a perception of the father as an object-thing, still almost an inanimate/extension of himself, one that is not autonomous, that dares to challenge the established and change place, "pretending" that he will not join them?

As Patrick is taken to his car, he alternately moves his look from checking his father's exit to staring at me, still inside the doorway. Are relevant processes of proto discrimination going on? A mirage, or real possibilities? There is no doubt that, on the sensorial apprehension level, a perception of differences takes place: the father who always leaves together, and the father who is indicating he will stay (this is strange and different!), the analyst who stays and the father who leaves (two distinct movements in relation to Patrick, which he compares by alternating his gaze).

In addition to the sensorial, even without knowing for certain what pre-existing elements there are at the representational level, we have seen more and more that one of the functions of our role is to attribute, to these children's perceptions, the intersubjective and humanised content. This repertoire, so present and banal in initial relationships, could remain absent or weak in autistic development. It is our aim to ensure that these expansions can be added to the child's emotional and relational repertoire (indeed, as well as to their neuropsychological and behavioural/social range). This is about an intimate, subtle, constant and almost minimalist experience of comings and goings, as our offer of humanisation doses can only be used or transformed in the measure and possibility of the given moment and the child's need. Is this not in itself an intersubjective experience, even if it involves aspects/nodes that are still autistic and crystallised? A mirage, or real possibilities?

What seems like a paradox, mirage or possibilities, can accompany our journey of expansion for what we consider as "mental" (usually associated with the "psychic" where there is more elaboration), to also include rudiments/proto-elements/primitive states of mind. In a visual flash allegory, the image of the mirage is part of the psychic nourishment needed by the person walking in the desert to reach the oasis, in the same manner that the good enough mother assumes/supposes the subject before the baby is fully there, and this anticipation is a bedrock for instituting subjectivity.

Final considerations: Facing the "black holes" and building up links

This clinical account illustrates the acknowledgement of gaps for establishing emotional contact based on minimal signs of communication, including expressions of well-being and discomfort, giving value to potential rudiments for bonds and self-other discrimination within autistic functioning.

With such pervasive disorders, the analytic approach is established by "pervading" crystallizing schemes for intrapsychic and intrafamiliar "pseudo-equilibrium", expanding the field of containment for the child, parents, families and the institutions involved in receiving and raising the rudiments/seeds/threads/incipient movements of recognition of oneself and other. These proto-bonding constructions are taken as foundations of intersubjectivity and allow for the expansion of the parents' and professionals' comprehension of the child's forms of functioning.

We evoked here the swings and continuous modulations that slowly and gradually allow professionals in the network to follow and facilitate the development of children with autistic disorders, including thinking and interventions that favour his genuine insertion into the family, school and social circles, with the potential achievements, impasses and suffering involved.

Returning to the allegory of the mirage, we must consider the resilience of the caregivers/analysts/seekers and the possible presence of the oasis/ areas of interest in the human elements, even if they are far away and threatened with being rendered useless if not reached in time. The autistic experience of the black hole (Tustin, 1981), as an area in which traditional physic laws cannot be applied, which is not really a hole, but whose existence can only be proved by the movement of the stars surrounding it (our countertransference), offers a live metaphor to further developments in psychoanalysis that might still come from detailed and clinically based investigations within this field.

With these ingredients, through building up links to process pains and human challenges, as well as facing the black holes in our patients, in ourselves, and in our psychoanalytic community, it is possible then to acquire new paths of development and psychic meaning.

References

Alvarez, A. 1992. *Live Company: Psychoanalytic Psychotherapy with Autistic, Borderline, Deprived and Abused Children*, London and New York: Tavistock/Routledge.

Alvarez, A. and Reid, S. *Autism and Personality—Findings from the Tavistock Autism Workshop*, London: Routledge, 1999.

Bion, W. 1962. *Learning from experience*, London: Karnac.

Barros, I.G. 2008. Explorações em Autismo. Trinta Anos Depois. Paper presented at the Paper presented at the International Congress: The Live Thinking of Donald Meltzer, 29-31 August 2008, São Paulo.

Barros, I.G. 2009. Para quem sabe ler, um pingo é uma letra. Paper presented at the National Congress of Psychoanalysis, May 2009, Rio de Janeiro.

Barros, I.G. 2011. Autismo e psicanálise no Brasil: História e desenvolvimentos. In: Schwartzman, J.S. and Araújo, C.A. (Eds). *Transtornos do Espectro do Autismo*. São Paulo: Memnon.

Ferro, A. 1995. *A técnica na psicanálise infantil*. Rio de Janeiro: Imago.

Haag, G. et al. 2008. Avaliação psicodinâmica de mudanças em crianças com autismo sob tratamento psicanalítico. In: *Livro Anual de Psicanálise*, Vol. XXI, pp. 137–153, São Paulo: Editora Escuta.

Lasnik-Penot, M.C. 1998. Psicanalistas que trabalham em saúde pública. *Pulsional Revista de Psicanálise*, year XIII, no. 132: 62–78.

Lasnik, M.C. 1995. *Rumo à Palavra –Três crianças autistas em psicanálise*. São Paulo: Escuta.

Lebovici, S. and Stoleru, S. 1983. *La mère, le nourrisson et le psychanalyste, les interactions prècoces*. Paris: Le Centurion.

Lebovici, S. 1986. À propos des consultations thérapeutiques. *Journal de Psychanalyse de l'Enfant*, 3: 135–152.

Lisondo, A. et al. 1996. Psicanálise de crianças: um terreno minado? *Revista Brasileira de Psicanálise*, 30(1).

Marucco, N.C. 2007. "Entre a recordação e o destino: A repetição", Conference at the Brazilian Psychoanalytic Society of São Paulo, March.

Mélega, M.P. and Mendes de Almeida, M. 2007. Echoes from overseas: Brazilian experiences in psychoanalytic observation, its developments and therapeutic interventions with parents and small children. In Pozzi-Monzo, M.E. and Tydeman, B. (Eds) *Innovations in Parent-Infant Psychotherapy*. (pp. 23–42). London: Karnac.

Meltzer, D. et al. 1975. *Explorations in Autism – A Psychoanalytical Study*. London: Clunie Press.

Mendes de Almeida, M. 2008. O Investimento desejante do analista frente a movimentos de afastamento e aproximação no trabalho com os transtornos autísticos: impasses e nuances. *Revista Latino-americana de Psicanálise*. Vol. 8/ 2008: 169–184.

Mendes de Almeida, M., Marconato, M.M. and Silva, M.C.P. 2004. Redes de sentido: evidência viva na intervenção precoce com pais e crianças. *Revista Brasileira de Psicanálise*, Vol. 38(3): 637–648.

Sherkow, S.P. 2008. Presentation at the International Symposium on Psychoanalysis and Autistic Spectrum Disorder, organised by The Margaret S. Mahler Psychiatric Research Foundation, New York, October 2008.

Silva, M.C.P. 2002. Um self sem berço. Relato de uma intervenção precoce na relação pais-bebê. In: *Revista Brasileira de Psicanálise*, 36(3): 541–565.

Silva, M.C.P., Mendes de Almeida, M. and Barros, I.G. 2011. O investimento subjetivante do analista na clínica dos transtornos autísticos. Cenas de uma intervenção conjunta pais-criança. In: Laznik and Cohen (Eds), *O bebê e seus intérpretes: clínica e pesquisa*. (pp. 205–215). São Paulo: Instituto Langage.

Sonzogno, M.C. and Mélega, M.P. (Eds). 2008. *O olhar e a escuta para compreender a primeira infância*. São Paulo: Casa do Psicólogo.

Spessoto, L.B. 2009. O sonho-alfa do analista como recurso para sustentação e desenvolvimento do continente e do conteúdo durante turbulência emocional. Paper presented at the Brazilian Psychoanalytic Society of São Paulo, April 2009.

Stern, D. 1985. *The interpersonal world of the infant*. New York: Basic Books.

Trevarthen, C. 2011. Desenvolvimento da intersubjetividade no primeiro ano de vida. In: Laznik and Cohen (Eds), *O bebê e seus intérpretes: clínica e pesquisa*. (pp. 117–126). São Paulo: Instituto Langage.

Tustin, F. 1981. *Estados Autísticos em Crianças*. Rio de Janeiro: Imago.

13 The Developmental Impact of Very Early Childhood on Treatment and Technique

Kerry Kelly Novick

Many colleagues have suggested that we are seeing new forms of psychopathology and that these demand evolution of our psychoanalytic techniques. I am not completely convinced that we are seeing new pathologies; rather, my impression is that symptomatology and presentation might have changed; fashions and labels in diagnosis might have changed; social and cultural values change over time, leading to new ideas about what is and is not normal or pathological. What feel unchanged to me are the underlying issues and conflicts that psychoanalysis is particularly designed to address.

That being said, however, I do think that there is always room for expansion and evolution of our techniques, to better meet patients and their families where they are and to offer the specifically individualised attention of the psychoanalytic approach. Here I will describe one direction in which I think we can enrich our understanding of what goes into technical choices and interventions.

The intellectual and emotional development of very young children before expressive speech is evident (0–27 months) resonates in many of our analytic techniques and can affect the trajectory of treatment in deep ways. In this note I hope to sketch some of those effects and suggest areas where we might direct further, more detailed, attention.

Modern developmental understanding places self-regulation in the centre of the organism's functioning. This maps very well on to psychoanalytic formulations, whether we look from the dynamic perspective, the economic, the structural, or the adaptive. Whichever theoretical model organises our individual thinking as clinicians we can share a general description of the goals and modus operandi of treatment in terms of helping the patient move to a place of being able to choose freely between predominantly neurotic or psychotic ways of regulating their experience and functioning and more adaptive, creative, and joyful modes. Jack Novick and I have described this in our model of two systems of self-regulation (2001, 2016).

In my experience, an interpretation often opens a doorway to new directions in the treatment, generates relief and a sense of "rightness" in both patient and analyst, and brings previously unconnected patterns into

DOI: 10.4324/9781003246749-13

juxtaposition with each other. But that is afterwards. There is also a pathway beforehand, that leads up to the interpretative moment, a series of steps that I think is grounded in a developmental line that begins in early infancy and mandates an optimal sequence for our technical interventions.

When babies are around four months old, parents begin pointing to objects, with their eyes, their voices and their fingers, and naming them. Babies at approximately six months start pointing, and adults usually answer the gesture with the word. By seven to eight months, a shared focus of attention becomes possible, with parent and baby looking together at a third thing outside themselves. By 11 to 13 months, reliable connections are established between things and their names and babies can use the symbol of the name or word to call attention and obtain what they want. Between eight and 13 months, the automatic equation of means and ends gets separated, and true cause-and-effect hypothesising begins. By 13 months, objects in the world (things and people) are perceived as independent entities, with their own properties, including the potential to be separate dynamic forces in the environment.

I suggest that we tap into the deep structure of this developmental line when we begin the journey toward an interpretation with patients of any age. First the analyst notices something and verbalises it—a feeling, a reaction, the use of a word. Then the patient also begins to notice it. Soon they are looking together at the phenomenon and wondering about it. One person or the other connects it with what usually precedes it or what it has been associated with. Together they puzzle over the nature of the connection. The analyst might then interpret how the connection arose and plays out in the present. Both patient and analyst can work together to clarify whether the original connection was accurate or represented the best hypothesis available to the child at the time.

Sometimes an interpretation falls flat. Perhaps it is just wrong and the analyst has missed something important. But here I would like to suggest that a failed interpretation might also result from skipping a step in the sequence described above. Each step has the potential to evoke defences when a person has suffered disruptions or interferences in smooth early development. Traumatic experiences demand the construction of defences, and these will be stronger and more monolithic the earlier the insult to the developing psyche. The accomplishment of each step in the sequence is necessary to make it safe to proceed further. Attention to this dimension might improve the precision and success of our efforts at interpretation.

All of this development and functioning takes place in the context of a relationship. Survival and growth of the infant, just like therapy, depend on the forming of a relationship. Here too I suggest that we can enrich our understanding of the therapeutic relationship by including attention to and knowledge of particular aspects of how the earliest relationships actually work.

I consider that the therapeutic relationship comprises four coexisting and interacting components: transference/countertransference, therapeutic alliance between both people and other parties to the treatment (parents, significant others), developmental object functions, and the real present interaction. These components show in different proportions at different moments and phases in the treatment, but it is important for us to keep them all in mind at all times, in order not to miss opportunities for authentic and effective interpretation.

Each component carries resonances of aspects of relationships experienced in infancy and toddlerhood. These can be characterised as the various experiences of self-with-other and conceptualised in relation to different types of interactions between infant and caregiver, each of which takes on subjective meaning for the infant along with the development of the capacity to experience the self as subject and agent. Classical descriptions of the psychic life of infants, whether framed as blissfully omnipotent and undifferentiated or as solipsistic inner dramas of hate and love among phantasy objects, seem to me to miss a more nuanced possibility of understanding the complexity of early development, which in turn produces the infinite variety of individual personality configurations we see in patients of all ages and the uniqueness of each analytic relationship.

Analysts, from Freud through Klein to Laplanche, have tended to describe attachment between infant and parent as mediated through drive gratification. A richer conceptualisation informed by the findings of decades of infant research suggests that attachment grows not only when babies experience ministrations (feeding, soothing, attention) that effectively transform their self-states, for instance, from hunger to satiation, or agitation to calm, but also needs additional experiences, described, for instance, by Stern (1985) as "state sharing" and "self-other complementarity". Lachman and Beebe (1993) place interpretation in this developmental context, proposing that the interpretive process involves all three aspects of the self-with-other, but privileging self-state transformations as the core of therapeutic action. Perhaps we can now specify these as appearing most clearly in the transference/countertransference dimensions of the relationship between patient and analyst.

State-sharing and complementarity might appear more essentially as elements of the formation and maintenance of the therapeutic alliance. Who the analyst actually is and what she offers to the patient in terms of tone, set, stance, and the framework of the treatment affect the developmental object and real components of the relationship they develop together.

There is another element from earliest childhood to take into consideration as we think about what colours and sets the overall tone of the therapeutic relationship. Parents who struggle to see their baby as a separate person usually have a very hard time in toddlerhood, as the child increasingly asserts her own wishes, desires, needs and aspirations. Many react to assertion as if it is an aggressive attack, with the twofold negative effect of creating mutual tension and hostility and defining for the child that wanting and achievement are aggressive. Analysts are also vulnerable to experiencing the separateness of the patient as a negative transference, an aggressive attack on the analyst or the treatment. It helps us when we stay aware of the deep developmental underpinnings of mutual and interactive experience, allowing us to respect the autonomy of our child, adolescent, or adult patients and working collaboratively with them to generate shared understandings. This is where we can see the interaction of transference components with alliance components.

Thinking about the developmental roots and resonances of our technical approaches and repertoire of interventions seems to me to offer the possibility of approaching new configurations of suffering and pathology with greater specificity and effectiveness, making it clear that psychoanalysis still has much to offer in the face of apparent social and psychological change.

References

Lachmann, F.M. and Beebe, B. 1993. Interpretation in a Developmental Perspective. *Progress in Self Psychology*, 9: 45–52.

Novick, J. and Novick, K.K. 2001. Two systems of self-regulation: Psychoanalytic approaches to the treatment of children and adolescents. *Journal of Psychoanalytic Social Work*, 8: 95–122.

Novick, J. and Novick, K.K. 2016. *Freedom To Choose: Two Systems of Self-Regulation*. New York: IPBooks.

Stern, D.N. 1985. *The Interpersonal World of the Infant: A View from Psychoanalysis and Developmental Psychology*. New York: Basic Books.

14 Video Child Psychotherapy During Lockdown for Better or for Worse

Julia-Flore Alibert

Keywords: Child psychotherapy, video sessions, tele-analysis, COVID-19, setting, transgression, collective trauma.

Lockdown

Following the home lockdown recommended by the health authorities from 16 March to 11 May 2020, I would like to share with you my experience as a child psychiatrist of eight weeks of video sessions with children from four to 15 years old. I see about 20 children a week for psychotherapy in my practice. I had to stop seeing my patients physically on Monday March 16 and suggested they all continue the sessions by video, Skype or WhatsApp. During that time, I was able to work in my office close to my home and the children could see me on screen in the room where I usually worked. The vast majority of patients agreed. The installation of the frame was initially a bit hasty. The situation was unprecedented. We didn't know how long it was going to last. I suggested that the parents leave the child in a quiet room alone with the phone in video mode.

The first week went by with great shared excitement. Children moving around with the phone, that's where the trouble started… most wanting to show me their things, their room, their bed, their toys, their blankets, the photos on the walls, their secret boxes… so far all has been going well, but some have gone so far as to show me their whole house: the brothers and sisters in their bedrooms, the living room, the toilets, the kitchen, and even…. the parents' room for primal scene! I was like snorkelling in their family intimacy … The camera on the phone is constantly moving, it gives me a headache, dizzy … but at the same time I find it interesting, I have the impression of seeing the world as them, as they want to show me. With these little cameramen I walk a meter high surrounded by giant objects … a table and chairs from this angle suddenly seem huge to me, I suddenly remember what it was like to be "small" surrounded by "Grown-ups" literally, the parents' faces are huge, the mouth of the one-year-old drooling sister gigantic, the family poodle looks like a lion!

DOI: 10.4324/9781003246749-14

Moving with their eyes, I became a child again, I reconnected more easily with my infantile part to better identify with them. Some young patients chose to draw calmly and show me their drawings, with others we try to invent games. With a five-year-old child we do a puppets fight: My cabinet puppets against his bedroom figurines. This makes possible to display great aggressiveness in this usually inhibited child. With others we play mime games, "rock leaf scissors" hand games, at the dinette everyone prepares their own dishes in their kitchen for a common meal, we even played hide and seek with a seven-year-old but I had trouble finding it when he left the screen! Those who could not isolate themselves in their room were in the living room or the kitchen and wanted to show me all the things that they are not allowed to do... turn on the oven, help themselves in the fridge and I had to tell them "no, don't stop touch!". Some wanted me to show them their file where I keep their drawings in the office, it reassured them to see that everything had remained in its place.

Phase of doubts

When the second week was over, I started to have doubts... what adventure had I started with them? How to maintain a therapeutic and exciting barrier in this worrying context of a global pandemic of indefinite duration... And how to work with this video tool which seemed to me at the same time interesting but also explosive and dangerous because it generates excitement and transgression. In the discussions with the groups of colleagues opinions were divided, some even preferred to give up and put the work on hold, while others continued to share experiences. This helped me to continue. Because spontaneously and with great simplicity, all my patients told me "see you next week" and they all wanted to continue the sessions, so I followed their movement. The parents were happy that everything did not end. They also told me how they managed daily life, teleworking with the children next door is complicated ... The first two weeks, most of the children were rather happy to stay at home with their parents than not to go to school.

Some have emotionally shown me their school workbooks, told me about their classmates who they already missed from their teacher. I was worried about those who could not isolate themselves at home, especially some teenagers who didn't want to continue the sessions remotely and whom I no longer saw.

Celestial: saved by the blue fairies!

From the third week of lockdown, the initial excitement subsided, and anxieties about the virus, death and disease appeared in the material of the children's sessions, in their drawings or their games. Children wandered less on the phone. A certain routine of the frame set in. It was the school break, the weight of the lack of freedom was felt even more. Global news was increasingly overwhelming. In my countertransference I was exhausted from these sessions which required extreme concentration. I had to take notes to remember from session to session, something I very rarely need to do. In each of my patients' pockets, where they usually store their drawings, I wrote down what they were doing behind the screen, to leave a trace. Some would notice and ask me "Why are you writing now? Are you afraid to forget? I was thinking… afraid to forget. This is not false." Working in my empty office was getting heavier and heavier, I missed the physical presence of my patients. We came to the end of the possible games to be played at a distance, sometimes a silence set in which you never knew if it was not due to a disconnection. Discouragement loomed over me. Personally affected in my close family circle by the virus, I was worried and working in these conditions was becoming more and more difficult.

I am going to bring you a piece of a clinical session with a little six-year-old patient from this period. Session of 1 April 2020. Céleste is a little boy that I have seen in weekly psychotherapy for almost a year. He had come for learning difficulties, a language delay taken care of in speech therapy, mutism and behavioural problems leading to relational isolation. He had a history of severe somatic problems in infancy that resulted in sensory isolation for several years. His parents had each gone through episodes of depression after his birth. A recent hospital check-up had diagnosed an attention disorder but no hyperactivity and recommended continuation of psychotherapy and speech therapy.

Before the beginning of the lockdown, Céleste had almost made up for all his academic delay and was doing much better. He had friends and even a sweetheart. The parents invested in their son's therapy and were in a good alliance with me. At the beginning of his therapy, in the sessions at my office, Celeste had repeatedly staged family stories where he played the role of a big brother with many responsibilities who had to take care of lots of household chores and help his parents. He found it hard to get out of this role and play freely, but he was more and more succeeding. At the start of the lockdown we agreed with his parents to do a video session on WhatsApp via a parent's phone: A new device for him and for me. The first two video sessions on WhatsApp, Celeste was installed in his room with the phone on his small desk, and he wanted to continue a card game he had made in the previous session at my office. I would show him his previous productions which I had kept in his cabinet pocket through the screen and he would continue to make other cards at home by drawing and cutting on sheets of paper. In the second video session, he was able to invent logical game rules and we were able to play his card game together. I was delighted to see a pleasure in logical and even mathematical reasoning emerge in this little boy whom we doubted the year before of the passage to the first grade. This is the third video session that I would like to present in more details because it is quite representative of the difficulties but also of the riches of continuing to work during the context of remote lockdown with children.

At the start of this video session Celeste is not very motivated, he does not know what to do and I offer to draw. I myself am in a rather gloomy mood overwhelmed by worries about the global health situation, on 1 April 2020 the epidemic curve was dizzyingly steep, and I was also reeling from bad news concerning my close family circle. Celeste starts to draw and shows me his drawing on the screen. I see a kind of big scribble in a circle. I ask him what it is, and he begins to tell me the next story that I am writing down. "It was a ball rolling on the road and after it fell on the magic clock. The magic clock has become stuck. She did not work anymore and now all the magic things didn't work anymore. All cars are blocked. All the people are no longer moving. Everything is at a red light. I ask him what this ball is and he continues. "It's a sticky ball who likes magic things, she comes back every end of the year, it eats everything, it gets bigger, bigger" I ask him if we can fight this ball and he replies "we tried a lot a lot for days, many days and it didn't work..." He looked discouraged at the time, and I too felt discouraged. The problem in his story seemed unsolved. Usually in these cases I always suggest that the child look for alternative solutions, but then I was overwhelmed by his discouragement. I still suggested without really believing "are you sure we can't do anything?" And Celeste remained silent and still behind the screen.

The silence lasted a while, I myself was plunged into a moment of discouragement, wondering if I should say something, but what ... I think we shared at that moment a silent moment of common depressive depression. I was myself invaded by very pessimistic fantasies of a world where it would be continually forbidden to move, travel, live freely, kiss friends and even bury the dead ... After a while time of silence, Celeste speaks "hello!" can you hear me there? "He walks over to his phone and speaks loudly to say" No... will work again!" I have an idea, I know what's going to happen. It's the fairies, the blue fairies! The blue fairies they will build a giant catapult, GIANT, I tell you, write it in capital letters! A giant catapult to get rid of the ball; they are going to have a lot of work but it will work. And the magic clock will work again and everything will work again! Celeste was very excited and happy as she said this. He starts drawing lots of blue guys all around the ball and shows them to me on the screen. He transmits his joy to me, and suddenly I feel like him, filled with joy.

I told him "Ah, what a good idea the blue fairies!" So we can say thank you and bravo to the blue fairies and the catapult, and everyone will be relieved when everything works again". It was the end of the session, see you next week. I turned off my phone, still feeling infused with his sudden joy and hope. In front of my black screen, I wondered what had happened during this session. In his story behind Celeste's blue fairies, I recognised the nurses he must have seen on television as heroines with their clogs, their charlottes and their blue paper coats in hospitals, and behind "the big ball that grows bigger and comes back to life every season "I saw the threatening shadow of the virus presented to the children in the form of a ball with spikes and finally in the catapult I saw a beautiful metaphor of the long-awaited vaccine which in a double movement first takes part of the virus for the better then get rid of it with the antibodies. In this session, on an emotional level, I got carried away in Celeste's story, going through with him a moment of common despair that we were able to overcome in a therapeutic way by following his final burst of creativity.

I tell myself that Celeste was very sensitive to my own depressive movement during the session. I myself was invaded at that time and independently of the Celestial session, by depressive movements linked to the disturbing news at the world level but also to bad news in the intimacy of my close family circle.

Celeste sensed this movement and it revived me a bit at the end with his creative impulse caught in manic excitement. Here he was replaying with me after the fact a movement he had already experienced with his parents who had gone through depressive moments in his early child-hood. Celeste came to my rescue, and I let myself be caught up, also saved by these blue fairies. I let myself be despaired by his story for a while, then I let myself be reached by his final joy and this sharing of emotion was a therapeutic experience for him. Taken as much as he was in the collective trauma that we both suffered, the difficulty was not to let myself be overwhelmed by my own depressive movement but to let myself be touched by his story without sinking into it. In this context of collective trauma, with my patient, I was caught up in the elements of realities and I used my own defences to overcome them.

In the next session, he wanted to continue his story, and we played together "kill the big ball with the blue fairies". With pencils stuck in front of the phone camera we made light sabres of all colours to deactivate the big ball. There was a lot of aggressiveness and cruelty in the material of the session in this little boy, who until then was rather inhibited in the session. Then he went to construction games he was making in front of me, making sure I was watch-ing him, jerky and fragile constructions that were becoming more and more ingenious and solid. Until then obedient enough for schoolwork at home with his parents, he opposed it more and more. Catching up on learning achieve-ments that had been difficult to achieve until then was again threatened. It was early May, the end of lockdown was looming, and I wrote to the school principal asking Celeste to be picked up as a priority. Celeste was able to return to school. In difficult conditions, he adapted to the new premises, to the new people, to the new rules. He resumed the sessions at the office.

It was touching to see each other again. We discussed the sessions on the phone again, the differences with the "live" sessions. "It's better to play anyway." We talked about disconnection problems: "sometimes you were on break, you moved more ... I had to wait". Also from the small size of the screen "when I moved too much, you couldn't see me more".

Today Celeste's treatment continues, I find him freer in his games. He let go of the role of big brother in his stories and lets himself go in his imaginary world and in games specific to his age. He will go to third grade.

This example of a child's cure with remote video sessions shows how much this new device has made it possible to continue therapeutic work while generating important technical questions about the setting.

Deployment of the cruelty of sadism

The video device with the telephone enabled certain inhibited children to display great aggressiveness in the sessions. Through the screen, some children were able to attack me more violently than they did in the presence, by threatening me with their toys ... bow arrows, sabres, pistols etc ... Some even took the phone to lock him up in their toy box. "I'll lock you up with my knights", a five-year-old boy told me and for a moment I found myself in the toy box with the unpleasant feeling of being immobilised like a turtle turned over on its shell unable to turn around. In this sense, the use of video is interesting because it can uncover unconscious, more archaic and more violent material. Like the dream, the video removes some censorship, and this can be a way of access to the unconscious. It is also seen in adults, the virtual world, the internet and social networks are the receptacles of all the aggressive or sexual gregarious impulses which are more easily deployed there.

Denial of separation and omnipotence

The use of video and remote sessions contributes to the denial of separation and to a certain fetishisation of the object. In this context, we did not know when we could meet again and how long the video sessions would last. Through the image of their therapist on the screen, some children were able to realise fantasies of mastery and omnipotence of the object by using and controlling the phone as they pleased. For some, it was necessary to take up during the reunion the differences between a person "in real life" and an image on a screen. A six-year-old boy told me at the reunion, "I liked it better when you were on the screen. Now in real life I can't take you everywhere, I can't turn you on and off". And even for parents, it was sometimes very practical to have the shrink at home, no need to travel, we can use it as we see fit. A parent at the end of a session, wanting to plan the next session and having picked up the phone, takes me to his room. Going to get his diary and putting the phone on the bed, he said to me "Doctor, I'm going to put you down there, I'm going to get my diary!"… and here I am in the very uncomfortable situation of waiting on his bed for him to come back …

Primary narcissism and exhibitionism

In video sessions, the child sees his own image on a small frame and by pressing on it he can make it big. Some kids had fun playing with it, they were mesmerised by their own image, and I could see they were looking at themselves on the screen throughout the shoot. A five-year-old boy spent a session like this admiring himself on the screen, imitating the speech of the French President, repeating in a jubilant and solemn tone "the schools will close until the new order!" Playing with the size of their image and mine was also a way for some of me to shrink and grow taller. "I made you small and me big!". However, for some uncomfortable teenagers, seeing themselves on the screen was unbearable and they preferred the sessions over the phone. For some children who did not look at the screen much and remained glued to their drawing sheet, I realised that it was especially difficult to confront their image. "I don't like to see myself". And for me, too, it was an opportunity to work on my relationship with my own image and I had to put up with seeing myself constantly during these video sessions, sometimes from not very flattering angles.

Privacy at risk

The device of the video sessions does not keep the privacy of the session as well as in the presence. Most of the parents respected the space of the session, but there were a lot of unfortunate intrusions that put me in uncomfortable situations … the cat, the little sister passing by, the notifications on the phone that interrupted the session. It has happened to me during the session that a parent was in the room but not in the field of vision, and with some it has been necessary to insist several times to preserve a private space. The brothers and sisters were able to see the session and some wanted to participate. Parents would tell me that siblings had fun playing outside of "Dr Alibert" sessions with each other. Some kids took advantage of having their parents' phone, which is usually off limits, to try to dig into their things, the phone book, or photos stored on the phone, and I had to tell them to stop.

Opposition and respect for the frame

In these conditions the respect of the frame was sometimes acrobatic. How to do a video session with an opposing child who deliberately leaves the field of vision? With a four-year-old girl having separation difficulties and unable to get away from her parents, we played hide and seek several sessions with her and her mother. And then gradually the mother was able to leave her alone with me. She hid outside the field of vision, then I asked her to show me a hand, a foot, an arm ... that she had fun putting in the field of vision of the phone, and then after that it was up to me. turn... back at the office, the child agreed to stay alone with me for a whole session, something she had never been able to do before. Another child was standing on purpose in the back of the room or from behind to prevent me from seeing him. It is then much more difficult than in the presence to interpret the passive opposition or to re-establish contact. For the child opponents who were more active in the transgression, it was also much more uncomfortable and difficult to get things back on track.

The lifting of phobic defences

For some children with social interaction disorders or social phobias, the remote sessions were paradoxically richer in material allowing a deployment of the internal world hitherto inaccessible. An 11-year-old girl, very inhibited with relationship difficulties, initially accepted the telephone sessions. She spoke very little the sessions were very poor. I offered the video to her and she set out to draw and invent a very rich and interesting story in which she was able to elaborate many of her internal issues that had hitherto been inaccessible.

Another 11-year-old with autism was very uncomfortable in the relationship in the face-to-face sessions, and he was much more comfortable with the video. He drew a lot and agreed to talk to me about his drawings in shared joint attention, while in the face-to-face session he locked himself in ritualised repetitive activities.

Reunion

The reunion after eight weeks was welcome, and it would have been difficult to hold out any longer. I had asked the children to create a pouch at home where they stored their session production. At the reunion they came with it, and we reassembled the two pockets. They showed me their drawings made during the video sessions and I showed them my notes. This allowed us to talk about the video sessions together and resume by putting into words what had happened. This reassembly process was important for the continuity of the work, to mark the difference and leave a trace of this exceptional period.

For better and for worse...

In the end, this experience of eight weeks of video sessions with the children during the lockdown was rewarding, even if at times exhausting. There were dark moments of discouragement when we had to hold out, cleared up by beautiful clinical moments. Despite the difficult and sometimes perilous conditions in which the frame was held, I believe that real therapeutic work was able to take place for the patients. The use of video has shaken the classical framework by its potential for transgression and deployment of infantile polymorphic perversions (sadism, voyeurism, exhibitionism) but also in some cases it has been able to reveal buried parts unconscious until then inaccessible. This was novel therapeutic work very different from the in person therapy of course, but therapeutic work all the same that we went through together... for better or for worse.

15 Working with Children and their Parents in Pandemic Times

Magdalena Calvo, Mónica Cardenal, Mariela Illán, Alicia Monserrat, Elizabeth Palacios and Andrea Souviron

Introduction

This presentation belongs to a set of them published in Spanish. All the clinical cases and theoretical thinking derived from a service designed in Madrid's Psychoanalytic Association to assist COVID-19 patients (couples, families, children and adolescents) and health care assistants during the Spanish confinement. We formed an agile group that responded to more than one hundred and thirty cases from eight public and private hospitals in the Community of Madrid, two healthcare centres, and some primary schools from Cantabria, Valencia, Bilbao Alicante and a community assistance programme from Zaragoza. The theoretical references and settings we usually work in our daily consultations had to be reformulated, being aware of the need to rethink our listening skills when assisting in an emergency. The full version of this study has been published by Psimática Editorial as *Psychoanalysis of Assistance in Emergency. Thinking the Pandemic* (2021).

The APM COVID-19 Commission began its work on 20 March 2020, with 79 professionals willing to give up working hours free of charge. An event that has produced and continues to produce effects, from which multiple meanings can derive, in an attempt to give figurability to the unrepresented aspects of this phenomenon. This event provoked our *deterritorialisation* (dislodgement), and that has made us move in search of new ways of doing psychoanalytically to achieve some kind of *reterritorialisation* (new lodging) (Deleuze, 2005).

The purpose of these reflections is to leave the trace of a period marked by the traumatic situation generated by the pandemic. COVID-19, the strange visitor, came to stay and remind us of human beings' vulnerability, pain, and helplessness. The interventions carried out through the APM COVID-19 Commission involved an innovative and challenging approach. It gave us the possibility of a transformation in our practice, and another type of mediation to help people who experimented psychic suffering. We have approached the needs of those who asked for help from our psychoanalytic listening but trying not to intervene in the latent and not to favour regression.

DOI: 10.4324/9781003246749-15

The work with children, adolescents, and parents has confronted us with the immediacy of events, the decline of everyday life, the surprise effect, and the fear of something unusual and unknown. The fear of contagion, death, and death without a last farewell, in the worst case, the loss of economic stability has provoked afflictions and despair for which we were not prepared, neither physically nor psychologically.

The confinement brought about a type of anguish in children and adolescents related to the conflict in the dynamics of their psyche: regression and progression as two poles of a line. The narrow family circle and the impoverishment of contacts with friends and other relatives justified in some children a regression imposed by external circumstances and revived childhood attitudes that had already been elaborated and had been overcome. We could observe a *traumatic progression mechanism* which manifests itself when young patients and children had to make an over-exertion, an early maturation to assume responsibilities for which they were not psychically prepared, consequently showing a pseudo-adult adaptive attitude related to controlling their emotions, balance, and repression of fantasies related to the COVID-19. The temporal dimension plays an essential role in this experience, as every human being needs time to process and assimilate the emotions that a trauma awakens in them. We had to help patients to process anxieties and put into words their emotions to facilitate our work as psychoanalysts, as well as, to cope with the mourning for the loss of a kind of life that was called into question.

We encountered conflicts at certain ages, as well as, in children and adolescents with great vitality and need for expansion. As we know, grief in this chronological framework is situated at an extreme ranging from separation anxiety to invasion anxiety. The pandemic has become a crossroads in the face of ambivalence in children and adolescents, between their desire for growth, personal progression, and their tendency to regress, now justified by events. This issue is confined to the family group, school institutions and the sociocultural context in which we are immersed.

Both in the consultations and the interventions of the COVID-19 device, we observed that the pandemic facilitated the unleashing and strengthening of inevitable conflicts that were compensated and in a latent state. We found the emergence of stories from the past, unresolved grief, and traumatisms that erupted like an erupting volcano through symptoms related to insomnia, hyper-excitement, paranoid fantasies, obsessive rituals and claustrophobia. This unprecedented situation swept away the previous established state and confronted us with an unparalleled feeling of helplessness, increasing and resignifying uncertainty. As psychoanalysts, we questioned ourselves when dealing with these crises, considering that during these months, the work with the children has been a great difficulty and the figure of the parents an essential element. Interventions online or by telephone, or through play, drawings, or verbal expressions have allowed us to mitigate the unconscious destructive and persecutory fantasies of contagion and death. The analyst is a mirror where the child will learn to discriminate between the adverse external reality and the replica of his inner life. Parents and the analyst are one of the supports on which the trust of children and adolescents is based.

If the confinement was traumatic, the deconfinement has highlighted other complex aspects to be taken into account. The refuge that the pandemic provided for the patients constituted an enchantment, a uterine fantasy for some of them that was not easy to transform. Some children and adolescents justified their refusal to go out for fear of becoming infected or infecting their family, but the unconscious motive was related to a regressive state in which they had settled. The danger that threatens the integrity of the self not only emanates from the intensity of the pubertal drives but also from the strength of the regressive impulse. This is how Peter Blos put it when he argued that the adolescent fears being trapped in infantile object relations.

Deconfinement has also highlighted the difficulties in elaborating mourning processes: a manic attitude, through massive outbursts, transgression of rules, attitudes of youthful euphoria, and denial of the illness. Unelaborated mourning is outlined as a shadow that hangs over all of us. A generalised sense of lust for life sweeps societies in the face of the threat of another confinement. Dissociative behaviours show how to live on two planes of existence: one, knowing the danger of contagion and its physical consequences and the consequences of economic chaos, and the other, living in parallel as if the threat did not exist. All the manic behaviours mentioned above show that confinement was an actual effort on a social level, but that in young people, it was an effort that was not fully integrated. As a result, a resurgence of the juvenile impulse was developed.

The reproaches from one generation to the other were intensified, and the universal grievances between the two are now exposed without repression. Young people faced the uncertainty of their future and felt immolated in the speculative ambition of the generations that preceded them. It is not surprising that *"presentism"* is a quality that prevails in the new generations as a reactive training that protects them from the anguish of the future.

Collaborating as a team in the COVID-19 Committee has allowed us to participate in clinical meetings where the interventions carried out were discussed. In the area of children and adolescents, two cases were presented by psychoanalysts from Madrid's Psychoanalytic Association, these were discussed by an invited psychoanalyst from Buenos Aires Psychoanalytic Association.

We hope that the uncertain experiences that the future holds for us can awaken our feelings of empathy and identify ourselves with other collectives and understand the dilemma of different generations; they will inherit a significant doubt about the future. In such difficult times as these, the transformative power of our psychoanalytic discipline must more than ever be at the service of society as a whole and, in particular of children and adolescents.

We must remember, elaborate, and not repeat, paraphrasing Freud, and recover the individual and collective memory that is often dormant. Eros must be above pain and despair.

First Clinical Case

"Where to point to?"

Through the COVID-19 programme organised by the APM, I have been following up with the parents of a child (especially the mother) who consult about their son Luis, who is currently five years old. It is the mother who gets in touch through the committee's email: "I am the mother of two children of similar ages. Luis is my son, and he has been sucking the index finger on his left hand since he was a baby; he is an active child. Since we have been at home, we have noticed he has started sucking it a lot more. We have tried various methods, but they have not worked. I would like you to give us some guidelines, so that I can follow them. He won't let us cover him up at night; calendars with rewards don't work?"

Once I received the referral from the coordinator, I contacted the mother by WhatsApp to arrange a telephone appointment. I received a quick response and heard a demand tinged with immediacy: she wanted it to be that same afternoon, in half an hour. I gave them the appointment as soon as I could and wondered what the urgency was. Both parents are professionals and have been teleworking throughout the confinement. The consultation was made when the father was back to work, and the children could start going out in a specific time slot. During this time, the mother told me that they had not been affected by any loss, owing to the coronavirus. During the first telephone interview, it is the mother the one who explains to me that Luis is a very "active" child: "He has not been a child who sucks his big toe, but his index finger. He has a deformed finger. He puts his finger in his mouth most of the time. We don't know what to do". Despite the concern they convey, I hear a contrast between the imminence with which they demand the first appointment and, on the other hand, the parsimony and lack of anguish with which they construct the story. The mother says that Luis has never stopped sucking his thumb, but of course, she says: "Being at school, we haven't seen it so much... now, it has surprised us, and we are even wondering if the school hasn't informed us".

They have been shocked by how repetitive this behaviour is throughout the day. She says that now he does it when he is calmer: when he watches cartoons on television or the tablet, and when he goes to sleep systematically every night. At this moment, the father is included in the conversation, who until then had not been present. The mother asks me if it is OK for the father to be included in the discussion, listen to me, and tell me (the most significant frictions in the house are with him). The father seems more anguished and powerless. He conveys his fears and frustration through his anger with his son: "His palate is going to be deformed, he already has a deformed finger, we will have to put braces on him...". She tells me that they have talked to him, that they have scolded him and even punished him, but that he does not stop. "We've tried everything, bandaging his finger, a sticker calendar, promising him something he likes... Come on, and if you do well, we'll give you a toy and nothing. He doesn't give a damn. When he gets up, the finger is dry". The father recounts how he goes to Luis's bed to remove his finger from his mouth at night. "Nothing helps. And of course, he's of an age. He's been sucking his thumb since he was a baby. He has this habit, and we don't know how to get rid of it" "He is not a child of dolls". They consulted their paediatrician for this reason, who told them it was a question of time, and told them to calm down, "In time he will grow out of it" The comparison with his other brother quickly appears, who "has always been very quick-witted, more mature. The other one has always been easier. No dummy, no dummy. The bike, the bike".

However, Luis has had a more challenging time with everything. I hear a very marked contrast between the brothers concerning the phallic-castrated, which we can observe how it is repeated in other pairs of brothers: where one would be the narcissistic representative of the ideal and the other, the representative of something linked to disappointment, to incompleteness. What place does Luis have in the parental phantasmatic? What does he become the depositary of? How has he been constituted?

The first thing that strikes me is the demand since it is an emergency device, and apparently, it is not a demand of these characteristics. So, I take it as a family emergent, fruit of the overflow of parental anguish, strengthened by this confinement situation, as it speaks of concern before this situation we are living through. Although I could not help thinking that the free consultation motivated the demand, I also thought that this request of help was full of frustration and impotence.

My first impression is that they are both overburdened. "Now, at least, we can start going out", says the mother. Where from, I thought that my intervention would deal first with listening and then provide an analytical act. I will not delve too much into their history to avoid a massive deployment, and for that reason, I felt a bit boxed in. This was also my first experience with this type of intervention, so I tried to be cautious. I base my intervention on listening to what they brought. They demanded a magic solution, something I should tell them so that Luis could stop sucking his thumb, so that they would not have to face the impotence and the narcissistic wound that this implied; they demanded a fast response.

A priori, I thought it would be a case for a referral to a child therapist, who could work on the phantasmatic aspects of the parents. What deficits or excesses have there been in Luis's internal constitution, how the triangulation was being articulated, what was happening with the paternal function. However, the first line was to contain these parents, explaining to them how children express their psychic suffering in this abnormal situation that we were all experiencing and that they, although small, are not unaware of what was happening around them. We see how behaviours perhaps linked to a more regressive functioning reappeared with more intensity because it is also their way of expressing it.

I transmitted to them that growth is something dynamic and that Luis will have to be observed. I talk to them about the involuntary nature of his behaviour (the mother had told me how the father started to scold him) and how sucking his thumb, despite being something regressive, perhaps more typical of an earlier period, surely helped him at this time to be calmer and more contained. Why hasn't Luis been able to give up his little finger? Why the index finger and not the big one? Is it a mechanism that isolated him, that calmed him down? What does the symptom tell us of his history with this oral hyper-excitement, of the encounter with the mother, with the vicissitudes of triangulation? How has Luis been able to go through all the renunciations and conquests, all losses and advantages in the first stages of life?

The next call came five days later. The mother seemed more relaxed, and the father was not on the phone. When I ask for him, the mother told me that he was on a work call. It did not seem like a good time for our call, so I offered the mother the possibility of meeting at another time when the father could be there. She replied that she did not care that there was no good time. She immediately told me to call her "tu" (Spanish colloquial way of addressing another person)", that she felt uncomfortable if a used the more formal pronoun "usted". I told her that "usted" came more naturally to me but that she could address me the way she wanted, using "tu" if she felt better that way. She insisted and I decided to do so. She told me that everything was still the same, that they had tried to put words to it, that they had offered him a little doll to sleep with but to no avail. "It's still the same", the mother repeated. "I have nothing new to tell you; everything remains the same, what we told you already". She told me once again that it is only at times when he is supposedly calmer. That he is too active a child. I listened to her, with the caution of not opening aspects that did not fall within the scope of what I thought would be an emergency intervention. I told her that they could ask for a proper assessment.

Considering the current circumstances, but without ignoring their concern, since it seemed that they had been restless and powerless for some time now and did not know how to help Luis, I told them that we could offer this assessment in our psychoanalytic society if they decided to as for more guidance in this regard. A little curtly, she replied that she would insist to her paediatrician to see if she could be referred to a psychologist if she deemed it necessary when all this was over. I felt that this intervention might have been hasty and that it might have raised more resistance, where perhaps there was already some. Towards the end of the call, Luis appeared in the background and got on the phone.

I heard a lively child with good language, answering questions that the mother asked him. He told me that he was OK. The mother intervened: "Tell her if you are a good or bad boy", to which he replied that what he likes is to jump on the armchairs. The mother, laughing, replied: "Yes, but mum won't let you...". He said goodbye and left, lively. Here, as in the consultation, I also felt the contrast between the child brought by the parents and the child who appears towards the end of the call. So, we said goodbye and agreed to get in touch again next week.

The following week I asked them when it would be convenient for them to meet. They did not reply to the first message, and after a few days, I wrote another one to which they replied: "Hello Andrea, it's complicated for me. But we're still fine... but as usual. Don't be in a hurry". Although I wrote a couple of times in the following weeks to close the intervention, after that message, I never heard anything more from them. Why doesn't the question about Luis' suffering appear? Can these parents give him a place as a subject? What does Luis "point to" with his little finger? What does it show that they cannot see? Where does it point to?

Second Clinical Case

"Eve, or the Forbidden Apple"

The intervention to be presented here deals with the case of an eight-year-old girl referred by the COVID Commission. The setting is different from the usual one. The interviews, lasting 45 minutes, are conducted via video call, and the number of interviews were limited to eight. The therapist had to contact the patient's parents.

In the first interview with the parents, they explained the reason for the consultation: the child refused to eat since she choked the previous week. Previously, she had been a child who ate everything and did very well. Now at certain times, when asked why she does not eat, she says she is afraid of choking. The choking was not particularly serious; she thought she remembered it was with a piece of hamburger, but since then, she had not eaten anymore. She had only had some yogurt or milk those days. Eva was very apprehensive. She had made some attempts to eat, but she would spit out the food and wipe her tongue. "I want to eat, but my instincts prevent me from doing so", she said on one occasion.

Her parents described her as very cheerful, sociable, and family-oriented. She was in the third year of primary school and was a bit lazy but did well in her studies. She liked to read a lot and was writing a book with a friend. That day she got angry with her homework and tore up the page she was writing on. She was particularly good at following the rules.

During that time, she had contact with friends and family. Going outside now that she could go out, she said it was a drag. The parents, both confined, had been at home during all that time. A friend of the family who was a psychologist had recommended that they consulted a psychologist because he thought that this could be generalised anxiety. She sat down to eat and started crying. That morning she told us that the old Eva was trapped under the bed and could not get out. We acted out in our meeting that we were getting her out of that place.

When she was three or four years old, she had a recurring illness that she could not remember the name of. She got little red spots (Measles? Chickenpox? Rubella? Mumps?). None of those. But they could not remember the name. They had to look at her throat with a stick, and since then, she hates going to the doctor. She likes to play with babies, with tiny houses, with Nancy, and he wants to read a lot.

I explained to them the type of intervention that we would have and asked them to explain to the child who I was and that we would play and talk and, prepare the materials or toys she might need for our meeting.

First Meeting

I met a vivacious, friendly girl who quickly made contact.

E (EVA): Look, these are the toys I have prepared. Do you want me to show them to you?
A (ANALYST): Sure!

She shows me several books she is reading, her Nancy doll, a whiteboard.

E: Do you want me to draw something?
A: OK. (*She drew a little pig. It was a copy from the internet, as she explained to me later on.*)
E: And now I'm going to draw the world. You know my teacher is going to have a baby?
A: Did she tell you in the online class?
E: No, it's a secret. I'm the only one who knows. She called me to understand what was happening to me and told me the secret.

I asked her about the old Eva, and she says ashamedly:

E: Don't pay any attention; that was nonsense. It was only a play.
A: Your parents told me that you're afraid of choking.
E: Yes, I've choked twice, once eating a hamburger and once eating meat.

A: And you're afraid it will happen again, and you'll die?

E: No, it's not that.

A: Maybe it's that they'll have to take you to the doctor and stick the stick down your throat.

E: I hate that! When I was little, I had scarlet fever, and the doctor used to stick that stick down my throat, and I hate it, but I hate it, even more, when he looked at my pipsqueak.

A: He used to look at your piddle?

E: Yes, he used to make me like that. (*She made a gesture with two fingers as if to open.*)

A: And you hate that.

E: Yes, it's horrible!

The parents were very distressed and did not know what to do. I received a what's app from the mother asking me if they should take her to the paediatrician. I responded "no" and that I would call them the next day.

In the following interview, I had with the parents. I tried to contain them both, especially the mother who experimented great anxiety. She asked me again if she should go to the paediatrician and force her to eat. I suggested her not to do so, and that I did not see the need to visit the paediatrician. I even told them that an appointment with the paediatrician could be counterproductive. I suggested that they could offer her soft foods for the time being and that she could sit at the table with them and that they had to try to take the tension out of the situation. I also told them that I trusted that this situation would gradually resolve on its own if we could all be patient. I suggested that they could invite her to prepare the meal and above all, that they had to try to convey calmness to their daughter.

Second Meeting

Eva told me about one of the books she had shown me at the previous meeting, the book "Karina and Marina". She told me that there were many videos of Karina on the internet but that her mother would not let her watch them.

E: I'll tell you a secret, I saw them one night, and there is nothing scary about them. I don't know why she won't let me watch them. Karina has a dog called Chanel, and so do I.

A: Yes?

E: Look. (*She pulled out a pink stuffed dog.*) And this is my Chanel, she barks and walks, not very well because she's had an operation on his leg, but she's going to get better.

Instead of moving forward, the dog turn on itself. She told me that she thought that this had something to do with the batteries.

E: Poor thing, she can't walk. Today I ate a churro, and as nothing happened to me, I ate some spaghetti. Look, my mother gave me this diary with a key because I ate lunch.

A: So no one can open it.

E: Of course. When we were coming here, we saw a dead dog and my mother told me not to look at it, and then it turned out to be a stuffed animal. Do you want me to read my diary to you?

She began to read it:

E: First day: I choked, and I'm scared. I'm not talking about it. Another day: Today I ate a churro, I hadn't eaten churros for a long time, and I saw that nothing happened. I'm still a bit scared. I don't eat steak. I want to go to Master Chef Junior. Today I'm going to cook.

The little dog likes to be petted here and there. (She touched his head and his back.)

A: And somewhere else?

E: On her tummy, but if I touch her, she likes it. But he doesn't like to be touched on his bottom.

A: And the pussy?

E: Bitches don't have pussy.

A: Yes, they do too.

E: Well, neither her ass nor her pussy. She's outstanding.

A: She doesn't bite?

E: No, look, if I put my finger in her mouth, she sucks it.

A: And does she like it?

E: Yes.

A: But you don't.

E: No, not me, no. Do you want me to play Karina's song for you? Me too, I'd like to make videos like her and put them on Tik-Tok.

A: And what video would you make?

E: 24 hours spying on my parents. No, not that. Why don't you help me write a letter to Karina?

A: OK.

We decided that each of us would say one sentence, and that she would write them down:

E: Dear Karina: My name is Eva; some nights I dream about you, I dream I'm with you. Can you put me in one of your books? I would like that very much. (Here, we leave a space, and I will put a picture of me). I would also like to record a video in your house and, also a Tik-Tok on your account and mine. (Your home is fantastic: it has five rooms, a garage, everything.) Could you follow me on your account? I'm your number one fan. Can you pass me your WhatsApp number? Book 3 is my favourite. I hope you answer the letter. Lots of kisses. Your number one fan. (I like to sign like this, so they don't know my name). Makes a doodle.

Interview with Eva's Mother before our last Interview

The girl was already eating well, although there were some foods such as meat that she refused to eat. The mother feared that she could have a problem with anorexia because she was worried about her weight. When I asked her to clarify this concern, she says that Eva had said that she would like to be like her friend X, who did not have a belly.

She was seen happier and calmer. There was one conflicting issue with Eva: every night, she went to her parent's bed. This had always happened. Her father sometimes left her stay, her mother did not, and the girl complained that this was unfair. The mother was afraid, although she thought it could be silly to pay attention to these things, but she commented that Eva came twice to tell her in secret that she thought that she was pregnant. Although the first time she explained to her that this was not possible, and told to her about menstruation, soon after, she came back to her mentioning the same fear of being pregnant.

Last Meeting with Eva

E: *"It's our last day, what a pity, what if I'm like you?*
  A: *Psychologist?*
  E: *Yes.*
  A: *"And I come to see you?"*
  E: *"Yes, please wait, I'm going to change to the computer".*
  While she gets the computer on, she asked me if my house was excellent. She was typing on the computer.
  E: *"Well, OK. That's it. Let's see, what's your name? How old are you?"*
  A: *"Eight years old".*
  She looked at me in surprise.
  E: *"Oh, right! And what's your problem?"*
  A: *"I'm scared".*
  E: *"What are you afraid of?"*
  A: *"I don't know".*
  E: *"Of the dark?"*
  A: *"Yes, and I want to be with my parents".*
  E: *"Well, you don't have to care about that. You just leave a little light on".*

A: *"What if someone comes?"*

E: *"To kidnap you?"*

A: *"Yes"*.

E: *"Don't worry, with the door locked, they can't get in. And do you have any other problems?"*

A: *"I have another one, but…"*

E: *"Let's see, tell me"*.

A: *"I think I'm pregnant"*.

E: *"No, not that… Do you have a boyfriend?*

A: *"No, I don't"*. (Making a gesture showing that she is out of the game). *"But you do, don't you?"*

E: *"Well, if you don't have a boyfriend, you can't be pregnant"*.

A: *"No?"*

E: *"No. You and your boyfriend get naked, so if you don't have a boyfriend, then nothing. Besides, do you have your period?"*

A: *"What's that?"*

E: *"That you have blood coming out of your pussy, but that's OK, you just put a sanitary towel on, and that's it. Well, that's it, if you have any more problems, let me know"*. (Using again the same gesture than before to show that she was coming of the game) *"It's just that I saw something on the Internet that said: 'I'm one hundred percent sure you're pregnant and I got scared"*).

Conclusion

Although the psychotherapeutic treatment that could address Eva's problems would be desirable (and I recommended it to the parents), this brief intervention has been fruitful.

It has helped to unravel a knot of conflict that could have developed into a more severe problem. The child's psychic characteristics, her capacity for symbolisation and play, and her ability for transference to be installed quickly contributed to this.

Her symptomatology seems to have coincided with traumatic aspects that have been reactivated and resignified with choking and aspects of infantile sexuality and Oedipal elements that have not been elaborated. Eva shows interests that are more typical of a pubescent than a latent child. I do not think that this is an eating disorder, although the symptom might lead us to believe so. Instead, I understand it as a conflict related to infantile sexuality: displacement of her erogenous zones, from the genital to the oral, sexual curiosity and the fantasy of pregnancy.

The possibility of representation through words and play has allowed her to reach up to a certain degree of elaboration and has made possible a certain decrease in sexual arousal with the partial resolution of the symptom.

Clinical Discussion by Mónica Cardenal

Scenarios of COVID-19: Child Analysis

I would like to begin my remarks with the words of Martha Nussbaum, a contemporary philosopher, a graduate of New York University, with a doctorate from Harvard, where she still teaches. In her view, this global and pandemic crisis is "a time of learning and resolution". In her interview with the newspaper *La Nación*, on 6 September 2020, she suggests:
"Now we all have a time to think, a time that we did not expect to have; we must take advantage of it".

I agree with this idea. I tend to be naturally optimistic. A commission such as the one proposed by the Madrid Psychoanalytic Association, for assistance during the crisis generated by COVID-19, integrated with a second space, that of group reflection-supervision, with a third space of elaboration of the experience and the work carried out with scientific production linked to it runs in the lines suggested by Martha Nussbaum.

What is it like to be a child analyst in pandemic times and during isolation? From my experience in these difficult and painful times, I arrived at the understanding that it is a priority to accompany children and their families through the continuity of treatment or through limited interventions such as the ones shown in this chapter—putting our analytical device into action. High anxieties were identified in each family member from the beginning of the pandemic. These were maintained and even intensified as time has gone by and sized differently. I have observed a significant level of depression, both in the parents and in the children whose mental state I will refer to in this commentary. When I include these observations, I am thinking of the clinic and the observance of babies. The experience of observation in the family environment and at a distance gave us an interesting perspective on the mental states of each of the family members, without losing the focus on the baby and its attachments. Exhausted parents, depressed in many cases by the economic situation or other losses that this pandemic produced, and young children using manic defences, charged with excitement. I consider the observation of babies in the family setting a critical complement to broaden our understanding of the emotional world of the young child in times of isolation and pandemic, and in this way, it has helped me rethink our forms of intervention in the psychoanalytic clinic.

"One of the main functions of the family is to contain mental pain". These functions are linked to the possibility offered by parents with their capacity to understand, promote love and favour the development of the mature procedures of children's minds.

Jeanne Magagna, in a scientific event held between the Committee on Child and Adolescent Psychoanalysis (COCAP) of the International Psychoanalytic Association and the University Institute of the Italian Hospital of Buenos Aires, through the Tavistock Model Postgraduate Infant Observation Course that I direct (August 2020), reported that in England there is an essential increase of depression in adults and physical abuse of children, as well as the presence of eating disorders associated with trauma and violence. He added that this disruption of internal emotional balance in the UK has led to creating an emergency mental health fund.

Experiences such as those gathered in these emergency interventions that we are analysing will provide us with data and a specific framework for investigating what is happening to the quality of the family's mental functions in such critical times as we are living in the world. In this way, I have the impression that we are accompanying and supporting many families in times of fear and strange sufferings, owing to everyday life that has been lost and transformed. Therefore, I believe we are working to make children feel less lonely and isolated.

Luis, a five-year-old child

"About the Hurries"

"Don't hurry", says the mother to the analyst in charge of the telephone communication, an analyst who is in order of helping her and, also her family. Perhaps, we could anticipate that what is "rushed" is the type of intervention. Us analysts need to know that it might be "little" in the urgency and whom we are assisting to have only seven telephone or video call encounters. Therefore, we must be prepared to bear the "urgency", the need I would add, of those who are making a consultation knowing that they have a limited amount of time to display their desperation or fears. It is clearly expressed that in the face of the anxiety that the consultation period is coming to an end, the mother prefers to end it earlier than planned. "Don't hurry", she says to the analyst, and she, the mother, hurries to exclude her. Perhaps some of the same anxiety that the mother evidence has been felt or suffered by Luis, whom we know has been putting his index finger in his mouth since he was a baby.

Was that finger integrating support, not soft, but a tense, hard nipple-penis, which united his self in that hardness and tension? Of course, I think of Esther Bick's concepts of a second skin at this point, and I bring back an appreciation of Jeanne Magagna (COCAP) Conference organised in Buenos Aires (August 2020) that refers to the "language of the hands" in babies and young children: "Hands waving for help, fingers clenched for security, fingers stretched out with tension, soft movements…". It is essential to consider that it is not the same to bring the thumb to the mouth as the index finger, which can be integrating because of its hardness and at the same time give an account of intensely intrusive mechanisms. He sucks his finger with force, so much so that his palate has even been deformed according to his parents' report. He seems to be using a highly hostile projective identification with effects on the self and objects, internal and external. Most possibly, Luis feels that with his index finger in his mouth all the time, he is somehow intrusively inside his inner mother (projective identification in the internal object), thus achieving, in his fantasy, a unique and exclusive, controlled relationship. This is not possible for him in the external reality that he shares with his twin brother ever since. From a baby's point of view, he is so interested in this domination and control of the mother from within his self, that he is practically not interested in toys, although we do know that he likes to move around a lot, which can also be a support for the self, in this case through action. We could agree that if it were this state of mind that I have just described, the proposed intervention would not help the child. We would need time for the implementation of an analytical process that would promote mental growth, in which Luis could stop holding his index finger in his mouth to deform it and start to have an internal integrating object that would not only sustain him but also help him to elaborate the hostility and intrusions on his objects of love. A passage from the sensorial world to the mind takes time. The analyst detected something and suggested a referral, but the mother's level of anxiety did not allow time for this. I found it interesting that the child was somehow in contact with the analyst trying to help, which is vital to the analyst. Perhaps he could appreciate that contact and help beyond his mother's rush and demands for someone to solve the finger in the mouth issue already as if this could be achieved without thinking about a process. Hurries are not proper for a growing mind with a capacity to appreciate attachments.

Eva, an eight-year-old girl

"Fear of choking…"

In the emergency care consultation for COVID-19, the analyst meets a girl who has been refusing food for a few days and says that her "instincts" do not let her eat, "they stop me". Her parents report in the first interview that there was an incident a few days ago in which the girl choked while eating a hamburger, a simple hamburger. That episode certainly only seems to be the trigger for blocking or claustrophobic anxieties: the child sits down to eat and starts crying, and one morning, she tells her parents that "the old Eve is trapped under the bed and can't get out". It is also evident that part of these anxieties is not being digested, not thought through in the child's mind. From that place, it is challenging to incorporate something that in the fantasy can be very destructive and get stuck, instead of promoting introjective processes or good incorporation experiences, which are the soothing tones of our inner world. This predominant state of mind occurs in a girl described by her parents as "very cheerful, sociable and familiar" perhaps at this time significantly affected by the situation of terror that the pandemic and isolation can provoke, conditions that intensify fantasies of violent intrusion: We also know that "she likes to play with babies, with little houses, with Nancy and, also likes reading". These undoubtedly more childish games seem not to be enough at the moment, to elaborate these more primitive anxieties, linked to claustrophobic experiences of being locked up in her oedipal objects, with the consequent return of intrusion upon her, with a predominance of oral fantasies. The interest in books seems to account for a more latent functioning. In any case, in the online sessions, the girl presents herself from the first moment eroticised and excited, where the defence turns out to be a hasty exit towards puberty as a way of calming the claims of polymorphous infantile sexuality as a state of mind (Meltzer, 1973).

I consider it essential to point out that the analyst, in her limited interventions in time, I am referring to the possibility of only seven calls, set the analytic device in motion. This is not a minor condition; this is how she suggests not to consult the paediatrician yet and enable this other framing option. From the analytical device, the child will unfold the anxieties and fantasies that she cannot digest and which, because of their strength and vitality, that of stories, she cannot swallow either. Thus, we enter the world of her books, of the things she hides from her parents at night, of the dead dogs, of the intimate diaries more typical of adolescent girls. In this way, the girl returns to eating, while in the meantime, she brings back to her encounters with the analyst, through the reading of her diary, her childish interests, conscious and unconscious: that the little dog "likes to be stroked here and there". (She touches her head and back). "But she doesn't like to be touched on her bottom". "Well, neither her bottom nor her pussy" (vagina). "She's outstanding"; "Doesn't she bite?" asks the analyst, "No, look, if I put my finger in her mouth, she sucks me off". "And does she like it?", "Yes", answers the girl. Eva tells us that she idealises an outstanding singer, Karina and that she would like to make videos like her and put them on "Tik Tok" "And what video would you make?" The analyst asks her.

In response to this, we have a very revealing answer: "24 hours spying on my parents. No, not that. Why don't you help me write a letter to Karina?" From then on, the girl begins to show her fascination with Karina, ambitioning her closeness by declaring herself her number one "fan", or rather "your secret fan", possibly of the analyst too, we would add. There appears an inner world hungry for pleasures that in her childish fantasy only adults enjoy; she ambitions that for herself, that is why she spies on the parents, she would spy on Karina and the analyst if she could. It is the mother who, towards the end of the intervention process, says that the child has always slept in bed with them. She presents herself as more assertive about this and sends her to her bed, but the father lets her stay.

Meanwhile, the girl says that it is unfair that they sleep together, and she has to sleep alone. There is something else that the mother reveals:

"Twice she told her very secretly and did not want her to tell her father that she thought she was pregnant". She explained to her, without going into too much detail, that this was impossible because women cannot have children until they have their period, a theme to which Eva returns insistently, and which she will even bring into her meetings with the analyst. It is there that she will unfold her emotional world, that of infantile sexual fantasy, where perhaps in a delayed way, or perhaps encouraged by the coexistence of the pandemic, (although we know that this child has slept with her parents since birth), the interests, curiosities, Oedipal intrusions vividly emerge. In the last interview, playing at being the analyst attending to her patient, or instead to her own projected infantile parts, she comments: "Well, if you don't have a boyfriend, you can't be pregnant". "You and your boyfriend have to get naked, so if you don't have a boyfriend, then nothing. Besides, do you have your period?"

These are Eva's interests which, because of the intensity with which they appear in her inner world, are unbearable and dangerous, so that they can drown her if they are not accepted and digested by an adult mind ready for the task, they cannot be thought by herself. Little Eva is desperate to understand the enormous curiosity and intrusive desires provoked by her parents' sexuality, which she lives as secret and forbidden to her, and now in an intense awareness produced by the pandemic, it excites her much more. It would be challenging for her to elaborate any of this with her parents because central issues of her childhood fantasy relate to them. Some of this was brought into play through the setting proposed by the analyst. Sleeping in her bed has not worked out well for her. She has not acquired much fundamental knowledge from it.

On the contrary, she has been trapped and drowned in her intrusion directed at the parental couple, with the consequent confusion and of zones inner spaces. The geographical disorders that should already be clearer and more ordered towards latency allow the mind to protect and delimit the areas that can accommodate babies productively and vitally (Meltzer, 1973). There are ways of knowing or perhaps not knowing (Bion, 1962) that choke and other proper forms of learning about sexuality help the mind grow into creative and fruitful inner states. In this way, the objects of love are left free, without the need to control them.

To conclude, if well carried out, the psychoanalytic method is a perfect tool, unique in its style, to promote emotional freedom and psychic growth, significantly affecting the quality of links (Cardenal, 2002). In global crises such as the one we are going through we confirm this even more.

My sincere thanks to the team of colleagues at the Madrid Psychoanalytic Association for inviting me to share spaces for reflection and clinical exchange, an experience that is always necessary for the progress of psychoanalysis and our work.

References

Bick, E. 1963. Notes on the observation of infants in the teaching of psychoanalysis. *APA Journal*, Vol. 24.

Bick, E. 1968. The Experience of the Skin in Early Object Relations. *International Journal of Psychoanalysis*, Vol. 49: 484.

Bion, W. 1962. *Learning from Experience*. Editorial Paidós, Buenos Aires.

Bion, W. 1967. *Returning to thinking*. Editorial Lumen, Buenos Aires.

Cardenal M. 2002. Object relationship vicissitudes: towards the acknowledgment of living dependency, young children observation. In: *Create Bonds*, Krakow.

Deleuze, G. 2005. *Lógica del sentido* (The Logic of Sense), Paidós, Mexico City.

Magagna, J. 2020. Conference "The emotional life of the baby in times of pandemic and lockdown", organised by the Committee on Child and Adolescent Psychoanalysis of the International Psychoanalytic Association, and the Infant Observation Course, Tavistock Method of London, given at the University Institute of the Italian Hospital, Buenos Aires, August 2020.

Meltzer, D. 1965. The relationship between anal masturbation and projective identification. *The Journal of Psychoanalysis*, 24(4): 791–808.

Meltzer, D. 1973. *The sexual states of mind*, Editorial Kargieman, Buenos Aires.

Index

Page numbers in **bold** refer to figures.

For Product Safety Concerns and Information please contact our EU representative GPSR@taylorandfrancis.com
Taylor & Francis Verlag GmbH, Kaufingerstraße 24, 80331 München, Germany

www.ingramcontent.com/pod-product-compliance
Lightning Source LLC
Chambersburg PA
CBHW060304220326
41598CB00027B/4234